Activity Analysis
Application to Occupation

FIFTH EDITION

Activity Analysis
Application to Occupation

FIFTH EDITION

Gayle I. Hersch, PhD, OTR
Associate Professor
School of Occupational Therapy
Texas Woman's University
Houston, Texas

Nancy K. Lamport, MS, OTR
Associate Professor Emerita
School of Health and Rehabilitation Sciences
Indiana University-Purdue University at Indianapolis
Indianapolis, Indiana

Margaret S. Coffey, MA, COTA, ROH
Activities Coordinator
Providence House
South Bend, Indiana

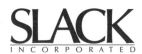

SLACK
INCORPORATED

An innovative information, education, and management company
6900 Grove Road • Thorofare, NJ 08086

ISBN-13: 9-781556-426766
ISBN-10: 1-55642-676-3

Printed in the United States of America.

Library of Congress Cataloging-in-Publication Data
Hersch, Gayle Ilene.
  Activity analysis : application to occupation / Gayle I. Hersch, Nancy K. Lamport, Margaret S. Coffey.-- 5th ed.
     p. ; cm.
  Rev. ed. of: Activity analysis & application.
  Lamport's name appears first on the previous edition.
  Includes bibliographical references and index.
  ISBN 1-55642-676-3 (alk. paper)
  1. Physical therapy--Handbooks, manuals, etc.
  [DNLM: 1. Occupational Therapy--methods. 2. Occupational Therapy--organization & administration. 3. Outcome and Process Assessment (Health Care)--organization & administration. 4. Task Performance and Analysis. WB 555 H571a 2005] I. Lamport, Nancy K., 1931- II. Coffey, Margaret S., 1950- III. Title.

RM735.3.L35 2005
615.8'515--dc22

                                        2004026375

Published by: SLACK Incorporated
                6900 Grove Road
                Thorofare, NJ 08086 USA
                Telephone: 856-848-1000
                Fax: 856-853-5991
                www.slackbooks.com

Last digit is print number: 10 9 8 7 6 5 4 3 2 1

CONTENTS

Acknowledgments . . . . *vii*
About the Authors . . . . *ix*
Preface . . . . *xi*

Module I   Activity: The Foundation of Occupation
Unit 1: The Impact of Occupation on Our Human Experience 5

Unit 2: Activity Analysis: The Learning Process 15

Module II   The Dimensions of Activity
Unit 3: Activity Awareness and Action Identification 35
        Form 1. Activity Awareness Form: Making a Telephone Call
        Form 2. Action Identification Form: Making a Telephone Call

Unit 4: Activity Analysis for Expected Performance 45
        Form 3. Activity Analysis for Expected Performance: Making a Telephone Call

Module III   Therapeutic Utilization of Activity
Unit 5: Activity Gradation and Adaptation 63

Unit 6: Activity Analysis for Therapeutic Intervention 73
        Form 4. Activity Analysis for Therapeutic Intervention: Making a Telephone Call

Unit 7: The Client-Activity Intervention Plan 85
        Form 5. Client-Activity Intervention Plan: Making a Telephone Call

Module IV   The Versatility of Activity
Unit 8: A Review of the Process 99
        Form 1. Activity Awareness Form: Making Cookies From a Recipe
        Form 2. Action Identification Form: Making Cookies From a Recipe
        Form 3. Activity Analysis for Expected Performance: Making Cookies From a Recipe
        Form 4. Activity Analysis for Therapeutic Intervention: Making Cookies From a Recipe
        Form 5. Client-Activity Intervention Plan: Making Cookies From a Recipe

Unit 9: Utilizing Assistive Technology: The Forms Web Site 123

Epilogue 125

Suggested Readings Prior to 1996 129
Suggested Readings From 1996 to 2003 135

Appendices
Appendix A: Position Papers of the American Occupational Therapy Association 141

Appendix B: Uniform Terminology for Reporting Occupational Therapy Services, First Edition 149

Appendix C: Blank Student Worksheets 157

Index *173*

Instructors: *Activity Analysis: Application to Occupation, Fifth Edition Instructor's Manual* is also available from SLACK Incorporated. Don't miss this important companion to *Activity Analysis: Application to Occupation, Fifth Edition*. To obtain the Instructor's Manual, please visit http://www.efacultylounge.com.

ACKNOWLEDGMENTS

We, the authors, again wish to acknowledge our colleagues, students, and families who have supported us in our long-term study of activity analysis as it applies to occupational therapy intervention. Our mutual history in this endeavor spans 20 years. We are especially grateful to our friends at SLACK Incorporated who have guided and nurtured us through four editions of this text and have encouraged us to complete still another. We are indebted to Franzina Coutinho, MAOT, a doctoral student in the School of Occupational Therapy at Texas Woman's University, Houston Center, for her literature search that updated our references.

We appreciate the opportunity to contribute to a profession that encourages us to grow professionally, intellectually, and personally. As coauthors, we are especially grateful to each other for the understanding and forbearance that we seemed to have maintained throughout every edition and still remain friends and colleagues. It is in this spirit that we dedicate the fifth edition of *Activity Analysis: Application to Occupation*.

Gayle I. Hersch, PhD, OTR
Nancy K. Lamport, MS, OTR
Margaret S. Coffey, MA, COTA, ROH

ABOUT THE AUTHORS

Gayle I. Hersch, PhD, OTR is an Associate Professor with the School of Occupational Therapy at Texas Woman's University. Her responsibilities are in the areas of teaching and research with master's and doctoral students. Her practice area is in gerontology with emphasis on Alzheimer's disease, stroke, caregiving, and home safety. Prior to joining the faculty at Texas Woman's University, she was a faculty member of the Department of Occupational Therapy, School of Health and Rehabilitation Sciences, Indiana University-Purdue University at Indianapolis (IUPUI)*, Indianapolis, IN.

Nancy K. Lamport, MS, OTR is an Associate Professor Emerita in the Department of Occupational Therapy, School of Health and Rehabilitation Sciences, IUPUI*, Indianapolis, IN. Prior to her retirement, her teaching responsibilities included fundamentals of occupational therapy (activity analysis), activities of daily living, leisure activities, and media. Her interests now include travel, community volunteering, and Medieval English tiles.

Margaret S. Coffey, MA, COTA, ROH is the Activities Coordinator of Providence House, an assisted-living facility for memory impaired adults in South Bend, IN. She is a contributing writer for *Spin-Off* magazine and teaches occupational therapy concepts in hand spinning and weaving activities to the well population. She is a former lecturer in the Department of Occupational Therapy, School of Health and Rehabilitation Sciences, IUPUI*, Indianapolis, IN.

* Formerly known as the Occupational Therapy Program, School of Allied Health Sciences, Indiana University School of Medicine, Indianapolis, Indiana.

PREFACE

This is the fifth edition of a book originally titled *The Activity Analysis Handbook*. This edition has been titled *Activity Analysis: Application to Occupation* to respond to the profession's focus on occupation as an approach to intervention. While the title and portions of the text have been updated, the content still reflects the ongoing growth in this essential area of our academic and professional knowledge base. When we began this work in 1983, instructional materials were drafted primarily to fill a void in class instruction. Forms were developed to bridge the gap in student learning regarding the importance and use of purposeful activity in occupational therapy.

As these forms have evolved, the intent has been to facilitate the student's understanding of what is involved in performing an activity and how the use of that activity can make a difference in a client's occupational performance. Regardless of the occupational therapy practitioner's frame of reference, theoretical background, or type of intervention, a thorough knowledge of activity and its application to occupation are required for credible and ethical practice. In this new edition, the authors continue to guide the student through the development of those clinical reasoning skills that are required to use and document purposeful activity in occupational performance. Whereas former editions of this text have been grounded by *Uniform Terminology*, the fifth edition is based on the principles of the *Occupational Therapy Practice Framework: Domain and Process* (American Occupational Therapy Association [AOTA], 2002).

As in previous editions, the text is divided into Modules and Units to facilitate the learning of more in-depth material in specific areas. There are additions and expansions to incorporate new information, clarify previously used material, and present relevant ideas that have emerged since the last revision. The references have also been updated. The overall structure of the five forms remains the same, but a significant number of the terms have been updated. The former Client-Activity Correlation (Form 5) has been retitled as the Client-Activity Intervention Plan. All of these forms are available on SLACK Incorporated's Web site (see Unit 9). The full or partially completed forms in the Instructor's Manual have also been updated.

The student should have ready access to the *Occupational Therapy Practice Framework: Domain and Process* (AOTA, 2002). This document is available for purchase from AOTA. It is also printed in the *American Journal of Occupational Therapy* (AOTA, 2002). Another valuable reference for the student is *The Guide to Occupational Therapy Practice* (Moyers, 1999), which was introduced as an additional way of focusing on the areas of practice and documentation.

Portions of *Uniform Terminology for Occupational Therapy I* (although officially rescinded) are included in Appendix A. It is retained for its historical value and as a resource for definitions of some of the terms used in Form 4, Activity Analysis for Therapeutic Intervention.

In this text, the term *practitioner* is used interchangeably with *therapist* as a simultaneous reference to both the occupational therapist and the occupational therapy assistant. In a similar manner, the term *intervention* is used in place of *treatment* or *therapy*. While these alternative terms facilitate our writing, we need to adhere to our roots. We are known as occupational therapists and occupational therapy assistants. Occupational therapy is our profession. We can value all of these terms as part of our professional communication.

References

American Occupational Therapy Association. Occupational therapy practice framework: Domain and process. *American Journal of Occupational Therapy, 56*, 609-639.

Moyers, P. A. (1999). The guide to occupational therapy practice. *American Journal of Occupational Therapy, 53*, 247-289.

Activity: The Foundation of Occupation

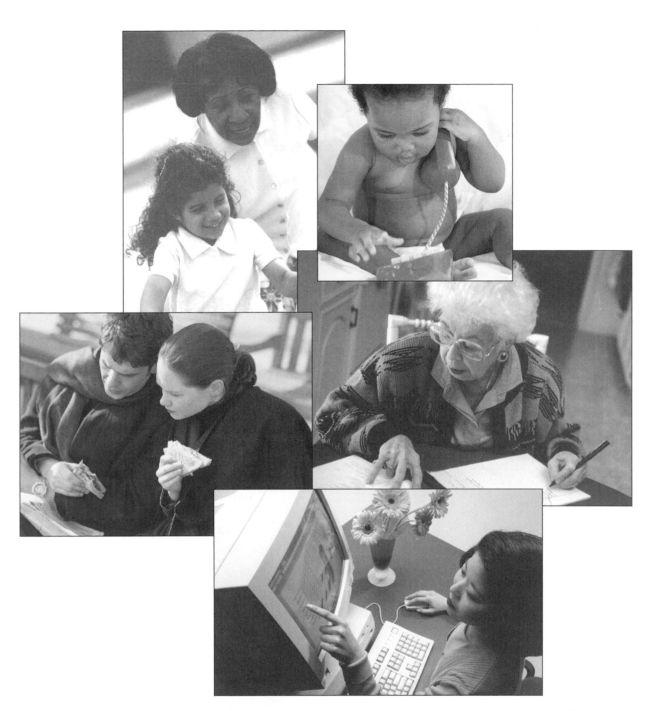

"Occupations are the ordinary and familiar things that people do every day."

Position Paper: Occupation (AOTA, 1995, p. 1015)

Unit 1

The Impact of Occupation on Our Human Experience

The human spirit of occupation, developed through eons of time in evolution, unfolding through development, and actualized through daily learning, needs to be nurtured to contribute to the health, quality of life, and survival of persons and society.

E. Yerxa, 1998

Historically, occupational therapy began with a focus on what people had to do despite illness or injury. This chapter will review the human need for meaningful occupation by examining the writings of selected recipients of the Eleanor Clarke Slagle Lectureships and other prominent writers of our profession. The impact of purposeful activity on occupation will be examined as the basis of intervention and the way it brings credibility to occupational performance.

OBJECTIVES

Upon completion of this unit, the student will be able to:

* Understand the vital relationship between occupation and quality of life.
* Recognize the importance of using meaningful everyday activities as the basis for intervention.
* Develop an appreciation of occupation as the philosophical root of occupational therapy.
* Consider the many ways that life roles can influence the client's occupational performance.

As human beings, we have an innate need to *do*. We build, we dismantle, we create, and we repair. We use tools and, if we don't have the appropriate tool at hand, we create one. We use and manipulate all forms of media, including space. We occupy our environment and we change it as our needs require. We are born with the curiosity to find out, to try, and to learn through all our cognitive and sensing mechanisms. We invent and then we reinvent. We nurture our progeny, our parents, our family members, and ourselves. We can reach out to offer support to people we don't even know and we can respond to people who reach out to us. We think, love, laugh, and live. We also pout, argue, and strike out. We have possessions, habits, traditions, and rituals with their significant signs and symbols, as well as laws and mores that provide meaningful attachments to our environment (Fidler & Velde, 1999).

We strive to achieve. We all know persons who have triumphed over seemingly impossible situations because of the innate need to do. At every age we try, make mistakes, problem solve, and try again. Sometimes, when we are overwhelmed with grief and despair, we realize that we cannot continue until we consciously decide to disengage and wait for our well of physical and mental resources to refill. A cup of coffee, a chat with friends or loved ones, a walk in the park, or a vacation can help us regroup. Sometimes we make the decision not to try again. What are the dynamics of our doing? We are living and consuming. Living is our occupation, and we are consuming the experiences of life. We can respond with spirit, optimism, hope, and faith in our environment and ourselves or be overshadowed by uncertainty, lack of enthusiasm, and, in some cases, despair.

The American Occupational Therapy Association (AOTA) (1995) writes, "Occupations are the ordinary and familiar things that people do every day" (p. 1015). In thinking about this definition of occupation, we realize that it has no confining levels of ability or disability. This realization provides avenues of intervention that were unrealized or unavailable when our profession was defined solely by the medical model. Now, with a resurging emphasis on the wholeness of occupation as the basis for practice, clients with or without disability can be served within the context of a facility, home, or community.

REALITY IN INTERVENTION

Each client referred to occupational therapy services brings a unique physical and psychosocial status, hopes and fears regarding present and future health, and the influence of significant others. All of these factors are embedded in the context of life experiences and are hinged, one with another. The performance skills that require attention are but a piece of the occupational competency puzzle. For example, a cognitive disability will impact not only a child's school-related activities but also all aspects of a child's life. The occupational therapy practitioner needs to develop an intervention plan that will enhance his or her total occupational performance.

The reality of occupation for any client is found within the home, the workplace, and the educational environment; with friends; and in the community. In choosing a real-life setting (e.g., the home) as the site of intervention, the practitioner accesses natural resources that can be utilized to enhance the client's occupational performance. By choosing selected elements of reality (or context), the intervention focuses on the center of that client's activity requirements.

Clark (1993) has described the therapeutic value of using true-life experiences as intervention strategies. Research has shown that contrived or nonrelated activity does not carry over into real-life situations (Thomas, 1996). Fisher (1998) outlines four of the commonly used methods of intervention seen in today's practice: exercise, contrived occupation, therapeutic occupation, and adaptive or compensatory occupation. She characterizes the first two as being therapist-imposed with no meaning or choice for the client. The third method of practice, therapeutic occupation, incorporates the issues of meaning and active participation by the client. The fourth method, adaptive or compensatory occupation, focuses on improving occupational performance through adaptive or remedial measures with no attempt to correct the impairment.

A real-life experience can call into play some of the remnants of former competencies that cannot be easily accessed in a mock-up situation. For example, an in-home kitchen experience can utilize the client's present assets, environment, and support systems in his or her natural setting. All the background nuances of familiar equipment, weight of utensils, counter height, sink depth, floor texture, ebb and flow of family and pets, fears of new experiences, and pleasures of success are present in an intervention experience that is couched in a natural setting. On-the-job training, learning to use an actual bus system, or taking care of a real baby brings reality to the intervention setting. Without these nuances of reality, the competencies noted when the activity is carried out in a clinical kitchen, a mock-up bus, or in diapering a life-size baby doll may not carry over into actual occupational performance.

INSIGHT FROM THE PROFESSIONAL LITERATURE

When we view all aspects of our lives as occupation, we acknowledge the precepts of thinkers and writers who have offered their philosophical research to illustrate the meaning and value of occupation as the foundation of our profession. Through his research on the persona of Eleanor Clarke Slagle, Bing (1997) offers a delightful insight into some of the origins of our developing philosophy that he presents as a scene of a play. The setting is Mrs. Slagle's kitchen in early December 1936. She is sharing some of her own history with three visiting occupational therapists. According to Bing, Mrs. Slagle insisted on using the term *occupational therapy* when speaking of this new profession. She felt that using only the initials "OT" was not informative enough for people to understand this new entity. Bing describes Mrs. Slagle's move to Chicago in 1911 and the beginning of her settlement work at Hull House. In 1912 she met Dr. Adolph Meyer who was developing his plan for the Henry Phipps Clinic at Johns Hopkins University in Baltimore. This clinic would house his new concept for treating the mentally ill, which he called an " occupational treatment center, a laboratory" (Bing, 1997, p. 224). He requested permission from Miss Lathrop, the director of Hull House, for Mrs. Slagle to come to Baltimore for 2 years to help develop this new clinic. Mrs. Slagle was excited to become a part of Dr. Meyer's vision for the care of mentally ill persons that would "provide support, encouragement, guidance, and a firm hand, when necessary, so a person could gain successes with occupations that had curative importance" (p. 224).

Later in the play, Mrs. Slagle further states her simple belief that occupational therapists "create situations, using the normal tools of everyday living, to maintain healthy conditions and a situation so that the afflicted individual can effect his own change, his own cure. Change occurs within the patient and we can only encourage it, modify it, and adapt it" (p. 226).

Friedland (1998) noted that emphasis was placed on the activity and the person during the early part of the 19th Century in both United States and Canada. The approach was not based on pathology (as with the medical model) "but on the interests and abilities and worked around the pathology to engage the person in occupation" (1998, p. 376). Friedland also noted that the need for rehabilitation services after World Wars I and II, followed by the entry of occupational therapy into the field of pediatrics, required an increased emphasis on personal independence and a decreased focus on occupation in the holistic sense.

Reilly in 1943 defined the difference at that time between occupational therapy and physical therapy when she wrote that "occupational therapy's purpose is to integrate the fundamental motions elicited by physical therapy into total activities" (Van Deusen, 1988, p. 146). Today, the focus of both professions has changed. Wood (1998) notes that physical therapy's present treatment practice is assuming a closer identification with occupational therapy's traditional goals of functional outcomes in work, self-care, leisure, and recreation (p. 404). She cites the need for occupational therapists to articulate the breadth and depth of our practice and research as "a historical progression of human services dedicated to everyday occupations as instruments of self-actualization, finding one's place in the culture, of realizing effective adaptations and experiencing wellness and health" (p. 408).

Miller, in her chapter on Kielhofner (Miller 1988) describes how he expanded upon the teaching of Reilly to develop the Model of Human Occupation. Clark (1993) and others developed the concepts of occupational science at the University of Southern California. Trombly (1993, 1995), Nelson (1996, 1997), Howard and Howard (1997), Baum and Law (1997), Gray (1998), and Yerxa (1997), as well as many others, wrote in support of the use of occupation as the foundation of our profession. Fisher (1998) described occupation as a noun of action that enables persons to do and to accomplish, while Christiansen (1999) used the concept of occupation as the key to identity, goal setting, and motivation.

In summary, the use of occupation as the focus for intervention brings the profession back to its roots and provides a solid identity that can be publicly explained and a unifying umbrella that covers all phases of practice. It is also important to recognize that there are those in our profession who view a basis for practice other than occupation (Pelczarski, 2000). Such an open debate provides a healthy venue for research and professional growth.

WHAT IS THE PARADIGM OF OCCUPATION?

There is discussion among the scholars regarding the significance of terms and how many (or few) entities comprise an occupation (AOTA, 1995, 1997). Not only is there discussion in the literature on how to use the terms *activity, task, occupational performance, function, functional outcomes,* and *intervention,* but how to sequence the use of these terms in a way that clearly demonstrates a client's progression toward occupational competence. When does a series of graded activities become an occupation? Can we assume that the occupation of lawn care is made up of a series of blocks of activity (i.e., planting, watering, weeding, pest control, and mowing,) nested together to form the construct of occupation? How does this construct differ for two clients when one is an elderly gardener with hip degeneration who diligently works in his bed of prized roses and the other is a professional nursery worker who sustained a rotator cuff injury from digging in heavy soil while gardening for a living? Were they not both engaging in their chosen version of the occupation of gardening?

If the questions above can be sorted into a logical and affirmative sequence, then we can conclude that each client has a personal set of blocks of activity that must be individually and carefully assembled to form the entity of gardening as occupation for that person. The number, size, and kind of blocks depend upon the purpose for occupational therapy intervention. For the elderly client, the reason is related to the need for leisure skills. For the professional gardener, the intervention is related to the role of work and productivity.

The terms *activities of daily living, work and productive activities,* and *play and leisure* are listed as performance areas in *Uniform Terminology III* (AOTA, 1994). For many years this document has provided the guideline for our professional communication and focuses on the use of a uniform descriptive language of our practice. In the previous text, the Performance Areas of Uniform Terminology served as a way of cataloging the occupations that are addressed when using purposeful activity as intervention. With the adoption of the *Occupational Therapy Practice Framework* (AOTA, 2002), our profession has taken a further step in energizing our areas of practice and clarifying our documentation.

THE SIGNIFICANCE OF ROLES

The first step in developing a meaningful intervention plan is to develop an occupational profile of the client. Trombly (1993) first suggested the practice of assessing from the top-down to gather a sense of the client's life role competence and meaningfulness as a way of clarifying the need for occupational therapy intervention. This differs from a bottom-up approach, which first focuses on skill deficits that may or may not hinder role function. Fisher (1998) proposed her Occupational Therapy Intervention Process Model as a top-down approach to evaluation and a framework for developing rationale and implementation of remedial and compensatory intervention.

As the client's life roles prior to the onset of disability are assessed, the following questions must be considered (Peloquin & Christiansen, 1997):

* What are the life roles of this client?
* Who are significant others, family members, or friends that comprise a support system and what is the status of this system?
* What is the client's work history?
* Is there evidence of community involvement or leisure activity?
* Has the client been successful, adequate, or marginal in these roles?
* What coping mechanisms, strategies for survival, and spiritual outlook on life are present?

Evaluation tools have been developed for gathering this information, and several current examples follow. Clark (1993) advocates the use of a life history, a narrative of the client's past. Fidler has developed the Interview Guide: Primary Occupation (Fidler, 1999). The Canadian Occupational Performance Measure (Law et al., 1994) is a third example. The client's historic occupational roles are as important to the intervention process as the evaluation of the disability. This information helps to develop an understanding of the client's occupational needs and must be an integral part of the initial evaluation. A thorough occupational history provides the compass from which to develop the direction and content of therapy. Costner (1988) states that occupational-centered assessments in pediatrics have not developed as readily as adult assessments due to the lack of a consistent framework. Trombly (1993) describes an adaptation of the functional assessment for adults to "better reflect the unique needs and situations of children" (p. 337). This previously little developed area of pediatric assessment has proliferated over the past 10 years. Asher (1996) cites multiple categories of pediatric assessment that include play assess-

ments, performance components, and infant and child development (neuromuscular/development) assessments.

The practitioner discerns what the disability means to the client and his or her caregivers through interview and evaluation, and discovers the human and environmental forces that are relevant to perceived life roles. The practitioner must look beyond the meticulously evaluated pathology to find the resources that can return the client to a meaningful role at home and in the community. When considering the client's status, it is necessary for the practitioner to guard against becoming so caught up in personal professional importance that the client's autonomy as a partner in the intervention process is overshadowed. Developing a mutual partnership leads to the trust and compliance that are necessary for successful practitioner–client therapeutic interaction.

THE ACTIVITY ANALYSIS AND CLIENT-ACTIVITY INTERVENTION PLAN

A beginning practitioner learns to analyze any human activity in terms of the human and nonhuman components that are required to fulfill its identity. This is the basis for activity analysis. Then, the value of that activity, used with a therapeutic purpose, becomes an intervention tool that can be applied to the client's context of life. This is a client-activity intervention plan. In the next unit, the student will learn to develop and use each part of the process of activity analysis and its application to occupational intervention. In a later unit, the student will learn to incorporate selected activities into strategies that will develop and implement occupational performance and to document the therapeutic outcomes.

DISCUSSION QUESTIONS

1. How has your concept of occupation changed following your reading assignment?
2. How does reality impact occupational intervention?
3. How does the role of the client influence the construct of occupation?
4. Which of your current roles is most meaningful to you and how does it fit into your present concept of occupation?
5. If your role as a student were to be compromised by a long-term illness, how would it change your concept of education as occupation?

REFERENCES

American Occupational Therapy Association. (1994). Uniform terminology for occupational therapy (3rd ed.). *American Journal of Occupational Therapy, 47,* 1047-1059.

American Occupational Therapy Association. (1995). Position paper: Occupation. *American Journal of Occupational Therapy, 49,* 1015-1018.

American Occupational Therapy Association. (1997). Statement—Fundamental concepts of occupational therapy: Occupation, purposeful activity, and function. *American Journal of Occupational Therapy, 51,* 864-865.

American Occupational Therapy Association. (2002). Occupational therapy practice framework: Domain and process. *American Journal of Occupational Therapy, 56,* 609-639.

Asher, I. E. (1996). *Occupational therapy assessment tools: An annotated index* (2nd ed.). Bethesda, MD: American Occupational Therapy Association.

Baum, C. M., & Law, M. (1997). Occupational therapy practice: Focusing on occupational performance. *American Journal of Occupational Therapy, 51,* 277-287..

Bing, R. K. (1997). "And teach agony to sing": An afternoon with Eleanor Clarke Slagle. *American Journal of Occupational Therapy, 51,* 221-225.

Christiansen, C. (1997). Acknowledging the spiritual dimension in occupational therapy practice. *American Journal of Occupational Therapy, 51,* 221-225.

Christiansen, C. (1999). Defining lives: Occupation as identity. An essay on competence, coherence, and the creation of meaning. *American Journal of Occupational Therapy, 53,* 547-558.

Clark, F. (1993). Occupation embedded in real life: Occupational science and occupational therapy. *American Journal of Occupational Therapy, 47,* 1067-1078.

Costner, W. (1998). Occupational-centered assessment for children. *American Journal of Occupational Therapy, 52,* 337-344).

Fidler, G. S., & Velde, B. P. (1999). *Activities: Reality and symbol.* Thorofare, NJ: SLACK Incorporated.

Fisher, A. (1998). Uniting practice and theory in an occupational framework. *American Journal of Occupational Therapy, 52,* 509-522.

Friedland, J. (1998). Occupational therapy and rehabilitation: An awkward alliance. *American Journal of Occupational Therapy, 52,* 373-380.

Gray, J. (1998). Putting occupation into practice: Occupation as ends, occupation as means. *American Journal of Occupational Therapy, 52,* 354-364.

Howard, B. S., & Howard, J. R. (1997). Occupation as a spiritual activity. *American Journal of Occupational Therapy, 51,* 181-185.

Law, M., Baptiste, S., Carswell, A., McColl, M. A., Polatajko, H., & Pollock, N. (1994). *Canadian Occupational Performance Measure* (2nd ed.). Toronto, Ontario: CAOT Publications.

Miller, R., & Keilhofner, G. (1988). In B. R. Miller, K. Stieg, F. M. Ludwig, S. D. Shortridge, & J. Van Deusen (Eds.), *Six perspectives on theory for the practice of occupational therapy.* Rockville, MD: Aspen.

Nelson, D. L. (1996). Therapeutic occupation: A definition. *American Journal of Occupational Therapy, 50,* 775-782.

Nelson, D. L. (1997). Why the profession of occupational therapy will flourish in the 21st century. *American Journal of Occupational Therapy, 51,* 775-782.

Neufeldt, G. (Ed.). (1997). *Webster's new world college dictionary* (3rd ed.). USA: Macmillan.

Peloquin S., & Christiansen, C. (1997). Occupation, spirituality, and life meaning (special issue). *American Journal Of Occupational Therapy, 51,* 167-168.

Pelczarski, M. (2000). Letters to the editor. We cannot hang our hat on occupation alone. *American Journal of Occupational Therapy, 54,* 112-113.

Thomas, J. (1996). Material-based, imagery-based, and rote exercise occupational forms: Effect on repetitions, heart rate, duration of performance, and self-perceived rest period in well elderly women. *American Journal of Occupational Therapy, 50,* 783-789.

Trombly, C. (1993). The issue is anticipating the future: Assessment of occupational function. *American Journal of Occupational Therapy, 47,* 253-257.

Trombly, C. (1995). Occupation: Purposefulness and meaningfulness as therapeutic mechanisms. *American Journal of Occupational Therapy, 49,* 960-972.

Van Deusen, J. (1988). Mary Reilly. In B. R. J. Miller, K. W. Sieg, F. M. Ludwig, S. D. Shortridge, & J. Van Deusen (Eds.), *Six perspectives on theory for the practice of occupational therapy* (pp. 143-167). Rockville, MD: Aspen.

Wood, W. (1998). Nationally speaking. Is it jump time for occupational therapy? *American Journal of Occupational Therapy, 52,* 403-409.

Yerxa, E. J. (1997). Health and the human spirit of occupation. *American Journal of Occupational Therapy, 52,* 412-418.

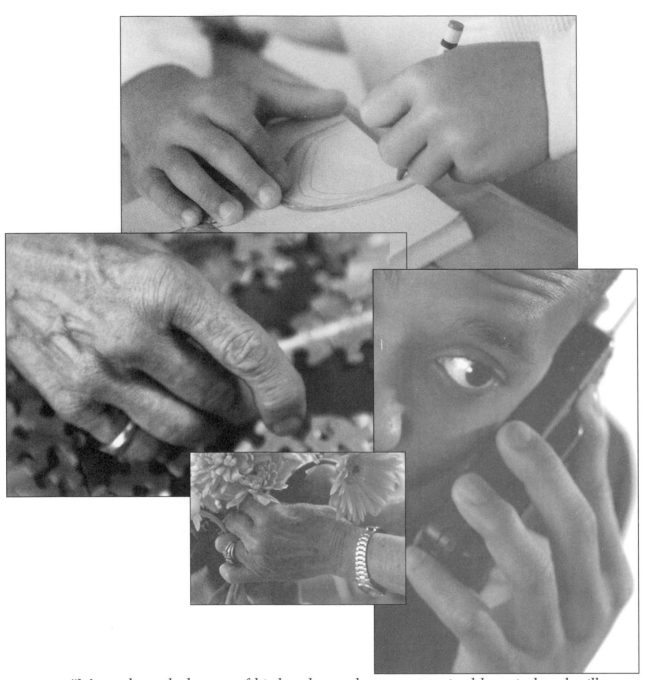

"Man, through the use of his hands, as they are energized by mind and will, can influence the state of his own health."

M. Reilly, 1962

NOTES

NOTES

NOTES

Unit 2

Activity Analysis: The Learning Process

OBJECTIVES

Upon completion of this unit, the student will be able to:

* Value the heritage of occupation and activity that is basic to the philosophy of occupational therapy.
* Associate the connections between occupation and activity.
* Describe the relationship between health and occupation.
* Recognize the way in which the *Occupational Therapy Practice Framework* can contribute to analyzing activity.
* Identify the role activity analysis plays in the clinical reasoning process.
* Apply the learning approach to activity analysis as presented in this text.

OUR HERITAGE OF OCCUPATION AND ACTIVITY

A reaffirmation of our heritage has taken place in the occupational therapy profession. The challenges presented by nontraditional media and other professional thinking during the 1950s through the 1980s reawakened the belief in and use of occupation in occupational therapy. Noted thinkers have summoned us to return to our roots, which date back to the early 1900s when the value of occupation was proclaimed, as noted by Reilly (1962) and

subsequently reaffirmed by West (1984), Fisher (1998), and Baum (2000). One of our founders, Adolph Meyer, recognized the value of work and occupation with his neuropsychiatric patients. In October, 1921, at the Fifth Annual Meeting of the National Society for the Promotion of Occupational Therapy (now the American Occupational Therapy Association), he stated that "the proper use of time in some helpful and gratifying activity appeared... a fundamental issue in the treatment of any... patient" (Meyer, 1922, p. 1). Upon reflection of his personal commitment to the use of activity in the psychosocial and physical treatment of patients, Meyer described this treatment as the "new scheme." In his words, therapeutic work "was a pleasure in achievement, a real pleasure in the use and activity of one's hands and muscles and a happy appreciation of time" (p. 3). Scattered throughout this historical writing are words like *performance, balance, actual doing, capacities,* and *interests*; words familiar to any contemporary occupational therapist and occupational therapy assistant.

Seventy-four years later, similar meanings of occupation were incorporated into the *Position Paper: Occupation* (AOTA, 1995a), "Occupations are the ordinary and familiar things that people do every day" (p. 1015). This simple definition captures the multidimensional and complex character of occupation. Reminiscent of Meyer's writings, major concepts embedded in the term *occupation* are that it be goal-directed, meaningful to the participant, extend over a period of time, and involve multiple activities (AOTA, 1995a). This multidimensional nature of occupation incorporates performance, contextual, temporal, psychological, social, and spiritual factors. Understanding and applying occupation to intervention programs for our clients becomes a challenge to the novice in occupational therapy.

As noted by Mosey (1986):

> *Purposeful activities cannot be designed for evaluation and intervention without analysis and synthesis. It is this tool that allows the occupational therapist to assess the client's need for intervention and to make a match between the interests and abilities of the client and the activities that will help to meet health needs, prevent dysfunction, maintain function, manage interfering behavior, and bring about growth and change.* (p. 242)

Consequently, an essential skill for any occupational therapist or occupational therapy assistant is to become proficient in the dual edge application of analysis and synthesis (i.e., "process of examining an activity to distinguish its component parts... and the process of combining component parts... to design an activity suitable for evaluation or intervention" [p. 242]).

OCCUPATION, PURPOSEFUL ACTIVITY, FUNCTION, AND HEALTH: TERMS AND CONNECTIONS

When the student begins to explore the heritage of our profession, a myriad of definitions and explanations of occupation, purposeful activity, and function surface from the literature (Christiansen & Baum, 1997; Moyers, 1999). Over the years, with variations in scope and length, explanations of these terms have emerged. Some terms like *occupation* and *activity* have been used interchangeably (Fidler & Velde, 1999); some theorists have proposed that a hierarchy of occupation exists and that activities are a subset. However, the reflective student will soon realize that regardless of the period of time or the author, a common thread is present: Occupation used in a purposeful and meaningful way can facilitate the health and well-being of the individual.

To clarify these terms, the Representative Assembly of the AOTA created and adopted several position papers. Beginning with "purposeful activity" in 1983 and later revised in 1993, this position paper makes a distinction between occupation and purposeful activity:

> *Occupation refers to active participation in self-maintenance, work, leisure, and play. Purposeful activity refers to goal-directed behaviors or tasks that comprise occupations. An activity is purposeful if the individual is an active voluntary participant and if the activity is directed toward a goal that the individual considers meaningful.* (p. 1081).

Webster's New World College Dictionary (1997) defines activity as "(1) the quality or state of being active: action; (2) energetic action, liveliness: alertness; (3) a normal function of the body or mind; (4) an active force; (5) any specific action or pursuit" (p. 14). Key meanings, then, are "active," "normal function," and "specific action or pursuit," all of which characterize the occupations most meaningful to the client and those in which participation is desired.

In 1995, two additional position papers were created and adopted, one defining occupation and the other defining function. *Position Paper: Occupation* (AOTA, 1995a) openly discussed the ambiguity over terms that has occurred over the years in the profession and acknowledged the multidimensional nature of occupation. Though recognizing that additional research and study were needed to fully understand this concept, the position paper did establish occupation as the hallmark of our practice. Prompted by the common use of function by other health care professions, *Position Paper: Function* (AOTA, 1995b) clarified the role of function in occupational therapy. It declared that function can be used "interchangeably with occupational performance because occupational therapy's domain is the function of the person in his or her occupational roles" (p. 1019). "Function" implies a comprehensive description of viewing the person performing activities and roles within a prescribed environment.

These terms were brought together in a cohesive manner with the 1999 *Definition of Occupational Therapy Practice for the AOTA Model Practice Act* (Moyers, 1999) adopted in 1999. This document explained that the practice of occupational therapy:

> *...means the therapeutic use of purposeful and meaningful occupations (goal-directed activities) to evaluate and treat individuals who have a disease or disorder, impairment, activity limitation, or participation restriction that interferes with their ability to function independently in daily life roles and to promote health and wellness.* (p. 608)

The "purpose" in purposeful activity is to elicit from the client a calculated response to the activity that addresses the identified intervention goals. Depending upon these goals, the performance of the activity may provide the means to increase strength, encourage social interaction, facilitate self-control, and/or stimulate cognitive integration. Activities may be graded, structured, or creative; they may facilitate prevention and/or adaptation. The key point is that as the client participates in purposeful and meaningful occupations, improved occupational performance becomes the outcome.

Ingrained in our history and as defined in the current Practice Act, occupational performance is integral to the promotion of health in the individual. Wilcock (1998) strongly makes this case by arguing two principles. One is that human beings have an "innate need to engage in occupation" (p. 22) not only to satisfy survival needs but also to stimulate and advance themselves. Human evolution is characterized by "ongoing and progressive doings" (p. 22). Secondly, engagement in occupation is intricately bound to complex health maintenance systems. Without involvement in activity, an imbalance and eventual decline of physical and mental mechanisms results (p. 29). These concepts are central to the philosophy supporting the value of meaningful occupational performance.

THE LANGUAGE OF OCCUPATIONAL THERAPY

Ultimately, the outcome of occupational therapy is to enable individuals to regain health through improved function in any occupations that are meaningful to them. Recognizing a need to convey this message in a succinct and universal language, our profession established a standard reporting system entitled *Uniform Terminology* (AOTA, 1979). The AOTA Representative Assembly adopted the first of these documents in 1979. It was later revised and adopted in 1989, and again in 1994 (see Appendix B for the first edition). This universal method of language was intended to be applicable for client documentation, reimbursement, and research. By having a common language, occupational therapists and occupational therapy assistants have the ability to communicate with each other, third-party payers, and other health care practitioners in a manner that greatly reduces communication discrepancies arising from subjective interpretation and unclear terms.

In 1999, the AOTA Commission on Practice determined that *Uniform Terminology III* needed to be revised due to the following reasons (AOTA, 1993):

* Changes in practice arenas
* The language being unclear to external audiences
* A renewed focus on occupation as the core of our profession
* Consensus within the profession that a change was needed

During this same period of time, the World Health Organization (WHO) reconfigured their *International Classification of Functioning, Disability, and Health* (ICIDH), emphasizing social and functional possibilities associated with health conditions, rather than pathology and limitations of disease. This new ICIDH-2 (WHO, 2001) focuses upon three dimensions of disability: the body level, including body functions and structures; the individual level covering the range of activities performed by an individual; and the societal level, or the extent to which an individual participates in life's opportunities.

The emphasis of this universal language upon activities and participation was recognized by our profession as congruent with the philosophy of occupational therapy. As a result of these concurrent influences, a revised language for practice evolved entitled the *Occupational Therapy Practice Framework: Domain and Process* (AOTA, 2002). Approved by the AOTA Representative Assembly, the purpose of this document is "to more clearly affirm and articulate occupational therapy's unique focus on occupation and daily life activities and the application of an intervention process that facilitates engagement in occupation to support participation in life" (p. 611). The domain part includes those areas in which occupational therapy provides service. The process part details the structural elements of the service delivered to the client.

Some of the language from *Uniform Terminology for Occupational Therapy—Third Edition* (UTIII) has been used and/or resorted into different categories. New language has been created, specifically performance patterns, activity demands, and client factors. A comparison of terms used in both the *UTIII* and the *Occupational Therapy Practice Framework* may be found on pages 637-639 of the *Occupational Therapy Practice Framework* (AOTA, 2002). In accordance with this, we have changed and updated our text to reflect the new *Occupational Therapy Practice Framework*. As one progresses through the activity analysis process, Forms 3 and 4 now reflect the language of the *Occupational Therapy Practice Framework*. We expect that further documents will be conceived and approved as our profession continues to evolve. Regardless of specific terms, the content of this text in learning how to think about activity in relation to occupation continues to be relevant in preparing future occupational therapists and occupational therapy assistants.

As a result of the new *Occupational Therapy Practice Framework*, a revision of the *Model Definition of Occupational Therapy Practice for the AOTA Model Practice Act* was drafted in October 2003 to reflect the new terminology and was brought to a vote at the AOTA Representative Assembly and approved in May 2004. We include it here so that the student will become familiar with this current definition:

> *...the therapeutic use of everyday life activities (occupations) with individuals or groups for the purpose of participation in roles and situations in home, school, workplace, community, and other settings. Occupational therapy services are provided for the purpose of promoting health and wellness and to those who have or are at risk for developing an illness, injury, disease, disorder, condition, impairment, disability, activity limitation, or participation restriction. Occupational therapy addresses the physical, cognitive, psychosocial, sensory, and other*

aspects of performance in a variety of contexts to support engagement in everyday life activities that affect health, well-being, and quality of life. (AOTA, 2004)

A DIAGRAMMATIC REPRESENTATION OF THE *OCCUPATIONAL THERAPY PRACTICE FRAMEWORK*

For educational purposes, three charts have been created to provide a diagrammatical representation of the activity analysis process incorporating the new language of the *Occupational Therapy Practice Framework* and represent our interpretation of the domain categories. The intent is to allow the student to visualize the entire picture of potential intervention outcomes and to distinguish each integral part of the activity analysis process. The three-page representation (Figures 2-1 to 2-3) depicts the interrelationships of the domain categories. Performance Areas and Skills, Client Factors, Performance Patterns, and Context are segmented into workable elements and then linked together to form potential intervention outcomes. The first illustration of the occupational performance chart (Figure 2-1) provides five major headings:

1. Performance in areas of occupation
2. Performance skills
3. Client factors
4. Performance patterns
5. Performance contexts

Figure 2-2 includes the major categories under each of the five major headings. Figure 2-3 illustrates the entire language of the domain part of the *Occupational Therapy Practice Framework*. In this way, one segment of the document may be studied and understood before proceeding to the next. In turn, the illustrations may assist the student in developing long-term and short-term goals by extracting the performance areas and skills that are needed to be addressed for a particular client.

As an example, examine the Performance Area of Occupation, Activities of Daily Living (ADL), which consists of eleven tasks:

1. Bathing/showering
2. Bowel and bladder management
3. Dressing
4. Eating
5. Feeding
6. Functional mobility
7. Personal device care
8. Personal hygiene and grooming
9. Sexual activity
10. Sleep/rest
11. Toilet hygiene

Within the performance area of ADL, the ability to dress may be differentiated into the three performance skills of motor, process, and communication/interaction and into client factors and performance patterns. Then, from each of these areas, specific components may be selected as applicable to client deficits. For example, motor considerations may be posture and coordination; process skills may involve knowledge and organizing space and objects; communication/interaction skills may include physicality and relations; and performance patterns of routine and role may be identified.

The major heading of performance contexts includes seven considerations. Any combination of these could have an impact on the client's engagement in the performance area of dressing. For example, the client's age, cultural background, and social supports could all have a bearing on the kinds of activities selected for intervention as well as those goals identified as most meaningful to the client.

Returning to the ADL performance area of dressing, two possible case scenarios are as follows:

1. A 72-year-old woman with a recent stroke and left side hemiparesis whose goal is to independently dress herself and attend her granddaughter's wedding but presents with left side neglect, weakness, and poor self-concept and lives alone in subsidized housing
2. A 15-year-old female admitted to an adolescent mental health unit for anorexia nervosa who presents with fatigue, negative self-concept, and poor attention to task

These cases are used to represent how intervention goals may be similar in outcome (i.e., improve dressing skills), yet differ considerably dependent upon the individual's circumstances or context. The occupational performance diagram serves as a template for potential outcomes, yet it allows for individual variation. The purpose of the charts is to provide the student with a diagrammatic portrayal of possible intervention considerations that promote occupational engagement.

RATIONALE FOR THE ACTIVITY ANALYSIS PROCESS

Since its founding in the early 1900s, occupational therapy has incorporated the process of activity analysis into its basic tools of practice. Creighton (1992) provides a rich chronological description of the inception of activity analysis into the profession. A detailed account is

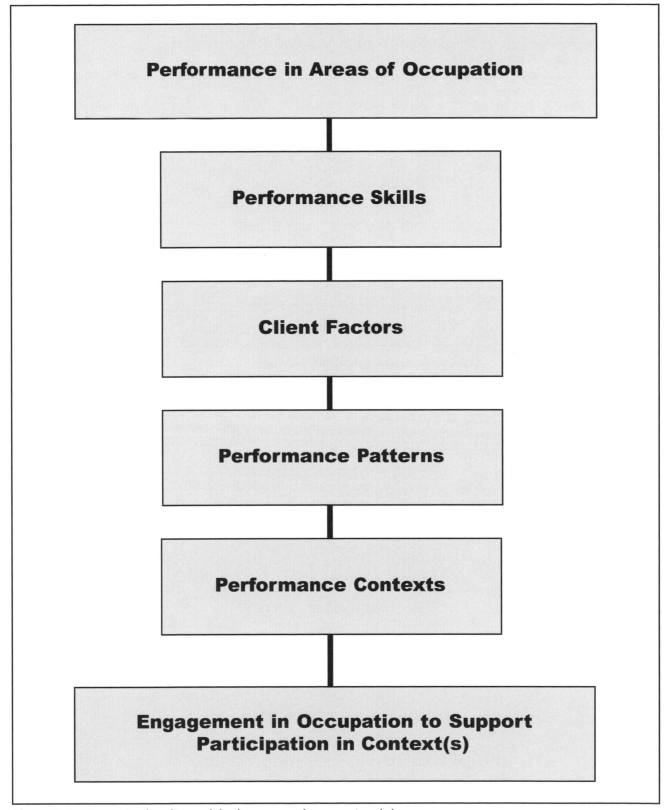

Figure 2-1. Five major headings of the language of occupational therapy.

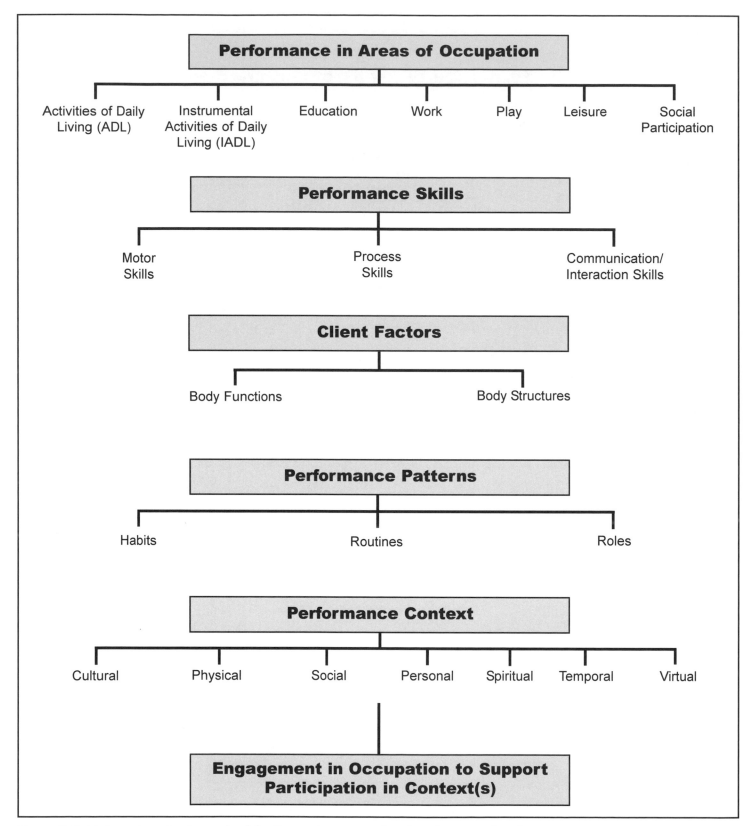

Figure 2-2. Major categories for each of the five major occupational performance headings.

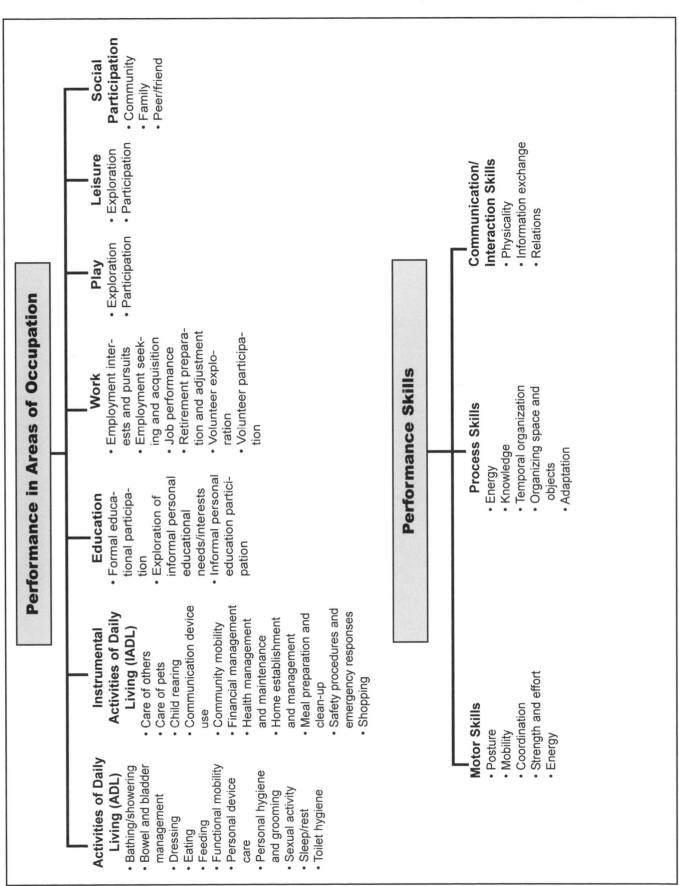

Performance in Areas of Occupation

Activities of Daily Living (ADL)
- Bathing/showering
- Bowel and bladder management
- Dressing
- Eating
- Feeding
- Functional mobility
- Personal device care
- Personal hygiene and grooming
- Sexual activity
- Sleep/rest
- Toilet hygiene

Instrumental Activities of Daily Living (IADL)
- Care of others
- Care of pets
- Child rearing
- Communication device use
- Community mobility
- Financial management
- Health management and maintenance
- Home establishment and management
- Meal preparation and clean-up
- Safety procedures and emergency responses
- Shopping

Education
- Formal educational participation
- Exploration of informal personal educational needs/interests
- Informal personal education participation

Work
- Employment interests and pursuits
- Employment seeking and acquisition
- Job performance
- Retirement preparation and adjustment
- Volunteer exploration
- Volunteer participation

Play
- Exploration
- Participation

Leisure
- Exploration
- Participation

Social Participation
- Community
- Family
- Peer/friend

Performance Skills

Motor Skills
- Posture
- Mobility
- Coordination
- Strength and effort
- Energy

Process Skills
- Energy
- Knowledge
- Temporal organization
- Organizing space and objects
- Adaptation

Communication/Interaction Skills
- Physicality
- Information exchange
- Relations

Figure 2-3. Descriptions of the five previous categories. (Adapted with permission from American Occupational Therapy Association. [2002] Occupational therapy practice framework: Domain and process. *American Journal of Occupational Therapy, 56(6),* 611.)

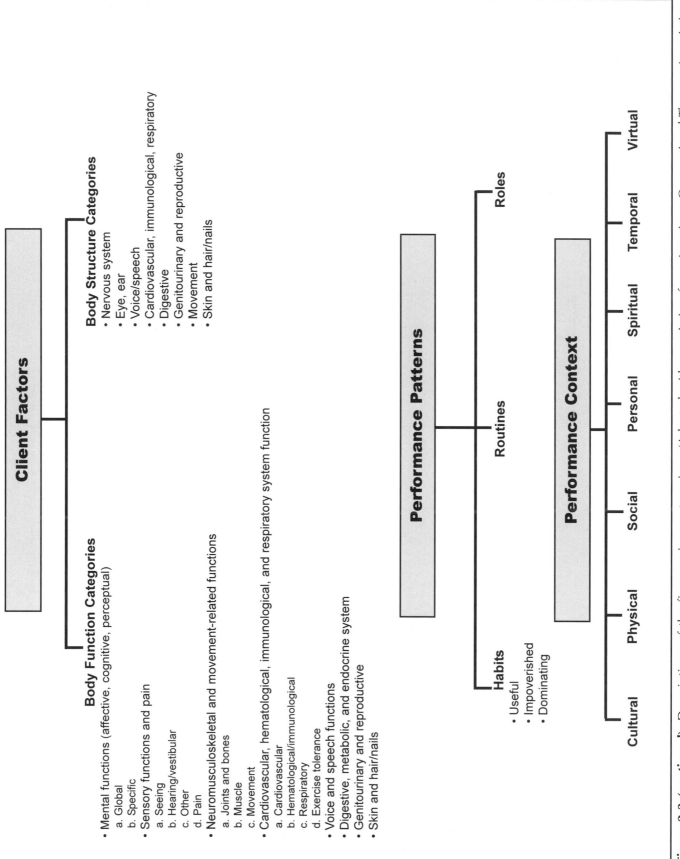

Figure 2-3 (continued). Descriptions of the five previous categories. (Adapted with permission from American Occupational Therapy Association. [2002]. Occupational therapy practice framework: Domain and process. *American Journal of Occupational Therapy, 56*(6), 611.)

given of writings by Gilbreth and Gilbreth dating back to 1911, 1920, and 1943, crediting their motion studies in business and industry and their training as mechanical engineers for the advent of "motion analysis" in occupational therapy. Over the years, the scope and depth of activity analysis has taken on many forms (Allen, 1987; Cynkin & Robinson, 1990; Haas, 1922; Licht, 1947; Llorens, 1973). Yet the core of activity analysis remains the same:

> ...*a process that assesses the elements or characteristics of an activity for the purpose of identifying and defining the dimensions of its performance requirements and its social and cultural significance and meanings. It is a process of looking at parts as these relate to defining the whole.* (Fidler & Velde, 1999, p. 48).

The key to intervention is the occupational therapist's and occupational therapy assistant's ability to analyze an activity and to make that match or synthesis (Mosey, 1986) with the needs and interests of the client. It is a skill that contributes to the clinical judgment and application of occupation in intervention. In turn, this ability determines the therapeutic effectiveness of the activity chosen. To be successful, activity analysis should be able to do the following:

* Provide a thorough understanding of the occupational performance of the activity and the knowledge base for instructing others to perform the activity.
* Contribute information regarding equipment, materials, cost, time, space, and staff to perform the activity in the therapy setting.
* Generate knowledge to judge for whom, when, where, and under what circumstances the use of the activity is potentially therapeutic.
* Detail the therapeutic benefits of the activity when used in the intervention process.
* Supply information useful in documenting an individual's progress in terms of the level of skill required or obtained, difficulties encountered, and reference points for intervention.
* Suggest alternative ways and means of performing the activity in an acceptable manner through modifying or grading the equipment, environment, and/or activity.
* Facilitate clinical reasoning in the selection of activities to meet the client's occupational needs.
* Provide a format from which to formulate intervention goals in any of the areas of performance for a given client.
* Encourage the use of the language of occupational therapy to describe, analyze, and document the use of activities that will enhance occupational performance.

THE LEARNING APPROACH FOR ACTIVITY ANALYSIS

Occupational therapy educational programs have been challenged by Yerxa (1998) to implement an occupation-centered curriculum that encourages self-directed scholars and generates an autonomous profession. Several concepts suggested for inclusion in this curriculum are grounded in the roots of our profession. One of those identified is activity analysis. The importance of "learning how to assess people's current ability in order to pose 'a just right challenge'... would be stressed" (1998, p. 370).

Taking this charge and implementing it into a meaningful learning experience for future students of occupational therapy presents a weighty challenge. Yet, it is one that is echoed about in many camps of the profession. The importance of occupation-based practice and the need for educating students and practitioners on the merits of returning to founding values of the profession to become well versed in the practice of occupational performance is reiterated by Baum (2000). Confirming our own beliefs as educators, the authors think it important to have a section on the justification of this learning approach to activity analysis included in this edition of the book.

It is our belief that the process of learning activity analysis follows a developmental path. The student acquires these skills over time in an evolutionary process. A certain mode of thinking culminates in the ability to see an activity and all its facets, and then matches those essential features with the client's needs. In many ways, this process is akin to the clinical reasoning process proposed by Mattingly and Fleming (1994). The assumption is made that clinical reasoning consists of three modes of thinking: procedural, interactive, and conditional. Mattingly and Fleming say, "In a procedural mode of reasoning, therapists search for techniques and procedures that can be brought to bear on the physical problem" (p. 119) and "interactive reasoning (is) used to help the therapists interact with and understand the person better" (p. 120). Conditional reasoning encompasses a greater sophistication and multidimensional art of practice seen most commonly with experienced therapists. In comparison, the analysis and synthesis of an activity can be likened to procedural and interactive reasoning. In that way, they serve as learned strategies that strengthen these modes of thinking.

The intent of this text, then, is to provide the student with a method of developing beginning clinical reasoning skills needed to identify, analyze, grade, and modify activities used in occupational therapy. In addition, activity analysis facilitates the thought processes involved in selecting activities for intervention and further clarifies how purposeful activities can meet specific client needs. To increase personal understanding of the inherent nature and therapeutic benefits of purposeful activity, students are encouraged to examine their own occupational performance and activities as part of this learning process.

The approach to learning activity analysis is multilevel. First, purposeful activity is examined in three different formats as it is normally performed. This process includes activity awareness, identification, and activity analysis. The activity is then analyzed according to its therapeutic qualities. Lastly, a specific activity or parts of an activity are matched or synthesized with a given client's intervention goals. Five forms are used to teach this multilevel approach and to help the student develop the thought processes required to apply purposeful activity to treatment. Understanding occupational performance and developing skill in using occupation therapeutically are essential features of an effective occupational therapist and occupational therapy assistant.

The five forms are designed to be used in a sequential manner linking the inherent characteristics of an activity with its therapeutic use. When this way of thinking about activity is applied, the analysis of activity becomes a conscious thought process. The forms are intended to progress the student from a basic understanding of the nature of the activity through the process of breaking it down into its components, and finally matching the therapeutic characteristics of the activity for client intervention. By using the forms, all the major facets of an activity are explored, and the skills required to engage in the activity are identified. Students are challenged to problem solve for alternative ways a client can perform an activity when skills are impaired or absent. They are also asked to describe how successful occupational engagement in an activity contributes to an individual's healthy lifestyle.

The authors believe that intervention outcomes should be observable, measurable, and subject to clear and accurate documentation. In this text, the *Occupational Therapy Practice Framework* and portions of *Uniform Terminology* are used as the basis for organizing and documenting the functional outcomes of therapy. Any activity used in intervention, no matter how complex, can be documented by using appropriate language. *Uniform Terminology* and the *Occupational Therapy Practice Framework* provide the student with definitions of terms that aid in describing activities and engagement in occupation.

In conclusion, developing the ability to analyze activities is perceived as a multilevel process, one step building on another. By using the forms to examine participation in a number of activities, the student experiences a wide array of avenues for analysis and synthesis. Upon completion of this textbook, the student is expected to feel competent in analyzing and applying activity that promotes a client's engagement in occupation.

Specifically, learning outcomes do the following:

* Identify the essential features of purposeful activity and occupation and the effect of activity engagement upon an individual.

* Describe the occupational performance of an activity in action step sequence.

* Analyze an activity in terms of occupational performance areas, skills, patterns, activity demands, client factors, and contexts.

* Identify precautions, contraindications, and acceptable criteria for completion of an activity.

* Formulate alternative means of performing an activity in an acceptable manner through modification of the activity or environment.

* Problem solve the selection of activities that meet the needs of a client receiving occupational therapy.

* Propose intervention outcomes that correspond to identified needs of the client in any of the areas of occupational performance.

* Apply appropriate language to describe, analyze, and document the use of activities in any practice arena within the domain of occupational therapy.

MULTILEVEL APPROACH TO ACTIVITY ANALYSIS

An occupational therapist and occupational therapy assistant examine an activity from at least two different perspectives: as it is typically performed and as a client may potentially perform it. Frequently, however, the practitioner must restructure an activity to place it within the client's range of abilities or use it to challenge the person to move forward in a performance area. Along with consideration of performance skills and patterns, client factors, and therapeutic implications, contextual factors impacting the client's life determine the choice of the activities used in the intervention process.

How, then, does the student organize all these elements into a manageable structure? Five forms have been developed to provide a template for gathering knowledge of all aspects of an activity and to establish a structure for learning. These forms should be used in the sequence in which they are presented until the student feels competent with them. The forms may then be used out of sequence to explore new activities or to approach a different understanding of familiar activities. The activity of "making a telephone call" illustrates all five forms. Blank copies of all the forms can be found in Appendix C.

Form 1: Activity Awareness

This first form provides an opportunity for an activity to be viewed subconsciously and highlights the student's personal response to a specific activity. The motor, cognitive, and psychosocial aspects of the activity are superficially identified.

Form 2: Action Identification

The second form provides a more direct approach to the actual performance of the activity. It separates the task into 10 or less sequential steps and also begins the process of observing variations of performing the same activity by several people in a Do-What-How format (Center for Learning Resources, 1979).

Form 3: Activity Analysis of Expected Performance

The third form provides an intense examination of the occupational performance areas, skills, patterns, client factors, and contexts of the activity. The student is asked to dissect the parts of the activity as it is normally performed, applying the *Occupational Therapy Practice Framework* terminology to describe its occupational nature.

Form 4: Activity Analysis for Therapeutic Intervention

In the fourth form, the student begins to consider what impact deficits or impairment of certain performance skills, patterns, client factors, and contexts may have upon occupational performance. Activity requirements, intervention implications, and modifications are to be delineated.

Form 5: Client-Activity Intervention Plan

The fifth form provides a structure for the application of an activity as an intervention strategy. The student is asked to complete a client profile including a description of the specific dysfunction from which long- and short-term goals of therapy are considered. The student suggests an activity that will be used as the intervention strategy, describes the preparation and implementation steps, and documents the functional outcomes.

SUMMARY

Occupational therapy practitioners need to use purposeful activity as part of their therapeutic intervention. The multilevel approach used in this text encourages the student to become aware of many different activities and their essential properties. It requires the student to break down activities into steps to identify the specific actions involved in performing them. It requires the student to examine the skills needed to perform those actions, as well as the context in which the activity takes place. Finally, it requires the student to look at a specific indi-

vidual's functional deficits and choose an activity that has meaning to the client and that will facilitate occupational performance. This educational approach is applicable to any activity used in occupational therapy and to any intervention setting.

DISCUSSION QUESTIONS

1. What is your understanding of our profession's heritage with activity and occupation?
2. Define activity and occupation and describe the relationship between these terms.
3. Explain activity analysis in your own words.
4. Identify the major categories of the *Occupational Therapy Practice Framework*. How has this document evolved?
5. What does the phrase "health through activity" mean to you as a future occupational therapist or occupational therapy assistant?

REFERENCES

Allen, C. K. (1987). Eleanor Clark Slagle Lecture. Activity: Occupational therapy's treatment method. *American Journal of Occupational Therapy, 41*, 563-575.

American Occupational Therapy Association. (1979). *Uniform terminology for reporting occupational therapy services.* Rockville, MD: Author.

American Occupational Therapy Association. (1993). Position paper: Purposeful activity. *American Journal of Occupational Therapy, 47*, 1081-1082.

American Occupational Therapy Association. (1993). *Uniform terminology for occupational therapy—Third edition.* Bethesda, MD: Author.

American Occupational Therapy Association. (1995a). Position paper: Occupation. *American Journal of Occupational Therapy, 49*, 1015-1018.

American Occupational Therapy Association. (1995b). Position paper: Function. *American Journal of Occupational Therapy, 49*, 1019-1020.

American Occupational Therapy Association. (2002). Occupational therapy practice framework: Domain and practice. *American Journal of Occupational Therapy, 56*(6), 609-639.

American Occupational Therapy Association. (2004). Definition of occupational therapy practice for the AOTA Model Practice Act, 58(6), 673-677.

Baum, C. (2000). Reinventing ourselves for the new millennium. *OT Practice,* (January 3), 12-15.

Center for Learning Resources. (1979). *T.A.S.K. A.C.T. A pre-instructional analysis process. Teaching improvement systems for health care educators.* Lexington, KY: University of Kentucky.

Christiansen, C., & Baum, C. (Eds.). (1997). *Occupational therapy: Enabling function and well-being* (2nd ed.). Thorofare, NJ: SLACK Incorporated.

Creighton, C. (1992). The origin and evolution of activity analysis. *American Journal of Occupational Therapy, 46,* 45-48.

Cynkin, S., & Robinson, A. M. (1990). *Occupational therapy and activities health: Toward health through activities.* Boston, MA: Little, Brown and Co.

Fidler, G. S., & Velde, B. P. (1999). *Activities: Reality and symbol.* Thorofare, NJ: SLACK Incorporated.

Fisher, A. (1998). Uniting practice and theory in an occupational framework. *American Journal of Occupational Therapy, 52*(7), 509-521.

Haas, L. J. (1922). Crafts adaptable to occupational needs: Their relative importance. *Archives of Occupational Therapy, 1,* 443-445.

Licht, S. (1947). Kinetic analysis of crafts and occupations. *Occupational Therapy and Rehabilitation, 26,* 75-78.

Llorens, L. (1973). Activity analysis for cognitive-perceptual-motor dysfunction. *American Journal of Occupational Therapy, 27,* 453-456.

Meyer. A. (1922). The philosophy of occupational therapy. *Archives of Occupational Therapy, 1,* 1-10.

Mattingly, C., & Fleming, M. H. (1994). *Clinical reasoning: Forms of inquiry in a therapeutic practice.* Philadelphia, PA: F. A. Davis Co.

Mosey, A.C. (1986). *Psychosocial components of occupational therapy.* New York, NY: Raven Press.

Moyers, P. A. (1999). The guide to occupational therapy practice [special issue]. *American Journal of Occupational Therapy, 53*(3), 247-322.

Reilly, M. (1962). Eleanor Clark Slagle Lectureship. Occupational therapy can be one of the great ideas of 20th century medicine. *American Journal of Occupational Therapy, 16,* 1-9.

Webster's New World College Dictionary (3rd ed.). (1997). New York, NY: Simon & Schuster, Inc.

West, W. A. (1984). A reaffirmed philosophy and practice of occupational therapy for the 1980s. *American Journal of Occupational Therapy, 38,* 15-23.

Wilcock, A. A. (1998). *An occupational perspective of health.* Thorofare, NJ: SLACK Incorporated.

World Health Organization. (2001). *International classification of functioning, disability, and health* (ICF). Geneva, Switzerland: Author.

Yerxa, E. J. (1998). Occupation: The keystone of a curriculum for a self-defined profession. *American Journal of Occupational Therapy, 52,* 365-372.

NOTES

NOTES

NOTES

NOTES

Module II

The Dimensions of Activity

Unit 3

Activity Awareness and Action Identification

OBJECTIVES

Upon completion of this unit, the student will be able to:

* Discern the relationship between activity and well-being.
* Become aware of hidden aspects of an activity.
* Identify action steps in performing an activity.

Activity has a dynamic quality that requires the individual to "actively" participate. The kind of participation varies with the activity, but this energy in doing is present in all activities undertaken. One way to define activity is "anything that requires mental processing of data, physical manipulation of objects, or directed movement may be considered an activity" (Trombly & Scott, 1983, p. 243). A more recent definition for the word *activity* is the "productive action required for development, maturation, and use of sensory, motor, social, psychological, and cognitive functions. Activity may be productive without yielding an object" (Christiansen & Baum, 1997, p. 591).

Throughout the lifespan, a person is engaged in activity. A great deal of being alive is just doing things. The decisions concerning what is to be done occupy considerable amounts of time as well. Based on the tasks set before the individual at any moment, activities appear to be selected that hold value and fulfill personal needs. In other words, activities take on significance and are done intentionally. As Adolph Meyer stated, "It is the use that we make of ourselves that gives the ultimate stamp to our every organ" (Meyer, 1922, p. 5).

In a real sense, activities are a vehicle for participating in life, for "being alive." From birth, the newborn engages in activity—looking, listening, learning. The process of doing becomes more complex as physical and mental abilities develop through childhood and adolescence. By young adulthood, the individual is increasingly involved in the "business" of life: meeting physical needs; attaining personal requirements; and participating as a member in society through school, work, or community responsibilities. Increasing awareness of how to accomplish these tasks in a way to elicit personal satisfaction develops with experience and maturation. Activities are not performed aimlessly but have a purpose or fulfill one. The individual begins to construct a lifestyle to provide feelings of efficacy, of joy in doing, and in affecting the personal world created (White, 1971, p. 274).

Because of the importance activities hold for humans, several underlying concepts regarding them are summarized as follows.

ASSUMPTIONS ABOUT ACTIVITIES

* Activities are primary agents for learning and exploration. Humans affect their world through doing, gaining pleasure and satisfaction through activities.
* Activities occur in normal growth and development. Engagement in activities is a part of being human and their intrinsic (built-in) value serves as a vehicle for healing.

* Activities have a potential greater than their surface appearance. Multiple areas of function are involved in performance that tap into a variety of body symptoms.

* Activities are a means of discovering one's self as well as a way of increasing function (i.e., "being" is embodied in doing). Individuals define much of who they are by what they do and choose to do (Fine, 1980).

Consider how activity is tied to health and well-being. When meaningful activity is not possible, the individual may become incompetent in meeting personal needs and performing developmental tasks. The sense of efficacy declines, and the challenge of life recedes for, in one sense, "to be alive is to have activities worth doing. When there are none, life is weary and worthless" (Reilly, 1977).

Thus a state of inactivity can indicate disability. When an individual loses the skills or ability to interact with the human and/or nonhuman environment, problems in "being," "doing," and "becoming" develop. Movement from one level of achievement and well-being to a lower one may occur. For example, the phrase "I'm not doing anything" has different shades of meaning depending on the person's perspective of wellness. This could signify temporary physical idleness, a mental state of reflection, availability or willingness to engage in activity, an emotional feeling of hopelessness, an actual inability to perform activity, all or none of these ideas.

Health is on a continuum, and the definition of being "sick" has a personal interpretation as well as medical one. When sick with a cold, the number and type of activities one is unable to perform is different than when one is sick with viral pneumonia. Similarly, coping with a broken arm is quite different than compensating for hemiparesis or an upper body amputation. In each of these instances, one is not necessarily "sicker" than another, but the optimum level of performance each person may achieve and the individual's perspective on what defines health is significant in influencing that person's sense of well-being. In short, the ability to engage in purposeful activity affects the quality of life. "The significance of engagement in activities and the value that such involvement has in sustaining health and a sense of well-being, in shaping quality of one's living and as a therapeutic and rehabilitative endeavor, is universally recognized" (Fidler & Velde, 1999, p. 6). There is a direct relationship between health and occupation (Christiansen & Baum, 1997, p. 14).

UNMASKING THE ACTIVITY: THE ACTIVITY AWARENESS FORM

Objective

Upon completion of the Activity Awareness Form, the student should be able to recognize the hidden facets of an activity as it is performed by a healthy person.

Understanding the inherent qualities of an activity is the beginning step to further analysis and therapeutic application for intervention. To dig beneath the surface appearance of what is happening in an activity can be as elusive as a dog trying to catch his tail. "A person who is involved in purposeful activity directs attention to the goal rather than to the processes required for achievement of the goal" (AOTA, 1993). The underlying side effects of performing activities must be identified by the practitioner to understand the connection between "doing" and "being," between occupation and health.

The intent of the Activity Awareness Form is to tap into the student's stream of consciousness to discover what occurs in the "doing" of an activity. While engaged, the student is unaware of what may be occurring other than what is apparent (e.g., opening a can of soup or sanding wood for a project). Through the use of the Activity Awareness Form, the student is directed to reflect on what is happening behind the scenes, to "catch in the act" the hidden aspects of the activity as it is performed. The focus shifts from the naming of what happened (e.g., "making a phone call") to what actually happens during the activity of "making a phone call" (see Form 1).

Directions

The student will perform the activity and, through use of the form, will:

* Recall the thoughts and feelings spontaneously evoked by the activity. These may include memories, desires, current concerns, or future hopes.

* Recognize general requirements of the body to perform the activity.

* Express cognitive, physical, or emotional stimulation experienced while doing the activity.

* Detect the ongoing effect of an activity after performance is completed.

* Identify a personal response to doing the activity.

IDENTIFYING THE COMPONENTS: THE ACTION IDENTIFICATION FORM

Objective

Upon completion, the student should be able to state major steps in performing a familiar activity in one sentence constructions.

As seen above, activities are more than they appear to be. Performing an activity requires the individual to use thinking processes, physical movements, and a variety of skills and functions. The next step in understanding the value of an activity is to distinguish the specific and sequential performance components of an activity from its general appearance. Looking at the major steps required to perform an activity helps to pinpoint the precise "action" taking place.

One method to describe action steps in objective terms is called the Do-What-How style. Based on materials from the Center for Learning Resource's *Teaching Improvement Project System for Health Care Educators (TIPS)*, each major step of an activity is described in a brief complete sentence. Steps are recorded sequentially beginning with a verb that indicates what to Do, followed by the specific action with What the person is to perform, and completed by a How phrase to clarify the verb and action (Center for Learning Resources, 1979, p. 15). Describing in words the actions taking place while doing an activity requires observing what happens on a performance level. Not only are the underlying elements of an activity unmasked, but close attention to the details of the "action" of the activity begins.

The significance of the direction (Do) and the action (What) may be more obvious than the descriptive qualities of the adverb (How). However, the adverb identifies the quality of the action required or observed as illustrated in the following: sit down slowly (a direction) vs. the client appeared to sit down slowly (an observation) (see Form 2).

Directions

The student will complete a simple activity and through the use of the form will:

* Identify and separate out major specific actions (10 or less) required to perform the activity.
* Record the steps in a Do-What-How sentence format.
* Observe and record someone else performing the same activity.

DISCUSSION QUESTIONS

1. What activities take up the most time in your life today, and how do these activities differ from those of a year ago? How do your activities differ from your classmate or your instructor?
2. Think of an activity that you derive great pleasure in doing and another activity you are required to do, but in which you take no pleasure. What makes one task enjoyable and the other disliked?
3. Briefly, what action steps comprise one of the above activities? What elements of the activity can you discern are "masked" or hidden beneath the surface appearance of "doing?"

REFERENCES

American Occupational Therapy Association. (1993). Position paper: Purposeful activity. *American Journal of Occupational Therapy, 47*, 1081-1082.

Center for Learning Resources. (1979). *T.A.S.K. A.C.T. A pre-instructional analysis process. Teaching improvement systems for health care educators*. Lexington, KY: University of Kentucky.

Christiansen, C., & Baum, C. (1997). *Occupational therapy: Enabling function and well-being* (2nd ed.). Thorofare, NJ: SLACK Incorporated.

Fidler, G. S., & Velde, B. P. (1999). *Activities: Reality and symbol*. Thorofare, NJ: SLACK Incorporated.

Fine, S. (1980). *The richness of activity*. AOTA Video.

Meyer, A. (1922). The philosophy of occupation therapy. *Archives of Occupational Therapy, 1*(1), 5.

Reilly, M. (1977). *Play as exploratory learning*. Beverly Hills, CA: Sage Publications.

Trombly, C. A., & Scott, A. D. (1983). *Occupational therapy for physical dysfunction*. Baltimore, MD: Williams & Wilkins.

White, R. (1971). The urge towards competence. *American Journal of Occupational Therapy, 25*(6), 271-280.

FORM 1
ACTIVITY AWARENESS FORM

Student: Example   Date:
Activity: Making a telephone call
Course:

Directions: Reflecting on the activity just performed, complete the following sentences with the first words that come to mind.

1. During this activity I was thinking about...

   All the things I need to get done today and hoping the person was home so that I could give her a message she needed before she left home.

2. While doing this activity I felt...

   Relieved when my friend answered the phone and I was able to talk to her.

3. In doing this activity, the parts of my body I remember using were...

   My leg while standing by the phone, my shoulder holding the phone against my ear, writing with my hand while she talked.

4. To do this activity I need to... (mentally, emotionally, physically)

   Remember her phone number, dial accurately, listen for the phone to ring, wait for my friend to respond, relay the information needed, and then replace the receiver.

5. When I do this activity again I will...

   Sit down after dialing the phone and have my list in front of me to check off items as I tell them to her.

6. From doing this activity I became aware of...

   How anxious I was to convey the message and complete this job on my list.

FORM 2
ACTION IDENTIFICATION FORM

Student: Example   Date:
Activity: Making a telephone call
Course:

Directions: Select an activity, and using the Do-What-How style, list the major actions in sequence in 10 steps or less required for you to perform this activity. Repeat the exercise after observing someone else perform the same activity.

Observation of Self

1. Open phone book deliberately.
2. Find number accurately.
3. Lift up receiver firmly.
4. Listen for dial tone carefully.
5. Push buttons appropriately.
6. Listen to other phone ring attentively.
7. Wait for response eagerly.
8. Say "hello" clearly.
9. Conduct and close conversation courteously.
10. Put receiver down securely.

Observation of Another

1. Find phone number carefully.
2. Pick up receiver confidently.
3. Listen for dial tone attentively.
4. Push numbers correctly.
5. Listen to ringing patiently.
6. Talk to person respectfully.
7. Cease conversation politely.
8. Hang up receiver firmly.

NOTES

NOTES

NOTES

NOTES

Unit 4

Activity Analysis for Expected Performance

OBJECTIVES

Upon completion of this unit, the student will be able to:

* Demonstrate a good working knowledge of the *Occupational Therapy Practice Framework* and apply it to activity analysis (AOTA, 2002).
* Analyze an activity as it would be expected to be performed.

ACTIVITY ANALYSIS FOR EXPECTED PERFORMANCE

According to Rogers (1982), the occupational therapy practitioner needs to have an in-depth understanding of the health-enhancing nature of occupation to use occupation or purposeful activity effectively in treatment. This understanding does not come about through reading or rote memory. It evolves from experiencing "normal" occupational performance and from knowing the therapeutic properties of occupation and the impact that performance deficits have upon occupation.

How, then, does this conceptualization of occupational performance occur? It involves a step-by-step dissection of an activity, whereby the student experiences the activity, uncovers the obvious, analyzes the skills required to perform the activity, and discovers its therapeutic characteristics. The intent of the Activity Analysis for Expected Performance Form (Form 3) is to provide the framework upon which this thought process of occupational performance could begin to develop. It is a systematic and comprehensive tool used to analyze a single activity.

An Overview

This third form is divided into four sections: Activity Summary, Analyzing Performance Areas of Occupation, Analyzing Performance Skills and Client Factors, and Analyzing Performance Patterns and Contexts.

Section 1: Activity Summary

Six areas of information are to be identified and described in this section and include the following:

1. Name and brief description of the activity.
2. Sequence of major steps and time requirements for each.
3. Precautions.
4. Special considerations such as age, educational requirements, and cultural and gender relevance.
5. Acceptable criteria for a completed activity.
6. Activity demands related to objects and their properties, including tools/equipment, materials/supplies, and space and social demands.

Section 2: Analyzing Performance Areas of Occupation

In this section, the dissection of the activity is studied according to seven broad areas of occupation. These performance areas are categories that are typically part of everyday life and include activities of daily living (ADL), instrumental activities of daily living (IADL), education, work, play, leisure, and social participation.

Section 3: Analyzing Performance Skills and Client Factors

There are two parts to this section: performance skills and client factors. Performance skills are basic human skills that are needed to successfully engage in the performance areas. Three aspects of the self emerge through these skills: the motor skills are the doing self, the process skills are the thinking self, and the communication/interaction skills are the feeling and social self (Crepeau, 1986). Client factors are those factors that reside within the client and that may affect performance in areas of occupation. They include body functions (i.e., the physiological aspect) and body structures (i.e., the anatomical aspect) of human performance.

Section 4: Analyzing Performance Patterns and Contexts

There are two parts to this section: performance patterns and performance contexts. Performance patterns are patterns of behavior related to daily life activities that include habits, routines, and roles. Contexts are factors that influence the client's engagement in the performance areas. They consist of cultural, physical, social, personal, spiritual, temporal, and virtual aspects of the client's world that have an impact upon the performance of the activity.

Objective

Upon completion of this form, the student will be able to describe an activity and provide the requirements to perform it as would be expected by a person with no occupational performance deficits.

Directions

To prepare for the completion of the form, the student should review the "Rationale and Learning Approach for the Activity Analysis Process" offered in Unit 2. There are four major sections of the form that should be completed according to the following guidelines.

Section 1: Activity Summary requires basic information about the activity. This information should be written in list or narrative form beside each item descriptor.

The student will do the following:

* Identify and briefly describe the activity.
* Identify the activity sequence and time requirements.
* Indicate the precautions and any other special considerations associated with performance of the activity.
* Provide acceptable criteria for the completed activity.

* Describe the activity requirements including objects and their properties and space and social demands.

Sections 2 to 4; Analyzing the occupational performance areas, skills, client factors, patterns, and contexts.

The student will do the following:

* Describe and analyze the activity using language conforming to current practice usage reflecting the domain of the *Occupational Therapy Practice Framework*.
* Examine the performance areas, skills, client factors, patterns and contexts of the activity as he or she performs it.

As an example, the student may be asked to address the performance area of ADL, and in particular, the task of brushing teeth. The student would provide a brief explanation by each of the categories needed to perform that grooming task. As the student proceeds through the list of categories, consideration should be given as to whether or not the category is applicable to complete the task as it is normally done.

Throughout the analysis, it is assumed that the student is performing the activity and the student's own expected responses should be identified, described, and reported. Keep in mind that only the actual performance of the activity described in Section 1 Activity Summary should be analyzed. For instance, if the activity is "brushing teeth," then the student may assume that the equipment and materials are gathered together at the sink area and are ready for the activity of brushing. The scope of the activity described in Section 1 determines the responses asked for in the other sections.

To illustrate an activity analysis according to Form 3, an example of making a telephone call is included. First and third person are provided in the form so that the student can see that an analysis can be addressed from different perspectives. Blank forms are available in Appendix C and on the Web site accompanying the text (see Unit 9).

DISCUSSION QUESTIONS

1. Identify the major categories for performance areas, skills, client factors, patterns, and contexts. What relationships can you make about the categories?
2. Why are you asked to describe the activity in Section 1 before beginning the analysis?
3. How did you feel as you analyzed an activity? What were you thinking?
4. How do you see activity analysis helping you later as a practicing clinician?

REFERENCES

American Occupational Therapy Association. (2002). Occupational therapy practice framework: Domain and process. *American Journal of Occupational Therapy, 56*(6), 609-639.

Crepeau, E. L. (1986). *Activity programming for the elderly.* Boston: Little, Brown & Co.

Rogers, J. C. (1982). The spirit of independence: The evolution of a philosophy. *American Journal of Occupational Therapy, 36*, 709-715.

FORM 3
ACTIVITY ANALYSIS FOR EXPECTED PERFORMANCE

Student: Example   Date:

Activity: Making a telephone call

Course:

Section 1: Activity Summary

Directions: Respond to the following in list format.

A. Name and Brief Description of Activity

   Making a telephone call from a desk telephone to a friend to confirm time to meet at movie theater. The student will prepare to make a telephone call, dial the number, convey a message to a friend, and close conversation.

B. Sequence of Major Steps (in 10 steps or less; specify time required to complete each step)

   1. *Sit in chair comfortably*   *3 sec.*
   2. *Find phone number in address book accurately*   *30 sec.*
   3. *Pick up receiver carefully*   *2 sec.*
   4. *Listen for dial tone attentively*   *2 sec.*
   5. *Press phone number correctly*   *10 sec.*
   6. *Wait for an answer patiently*   *7 sec.*
   7. *Talk to person clearly*   *15 min.*
   8. *Conclude conversation courteously*   *5 min.*
   9. *Put receiver down firmly*   *2 sec.*

   Total time = 21 minutes

C. Precautions (review "Sequence of Major Steps")

   The student should be aware of time restraints and may need to limit phone conversation.

D. Special Considerations (age appropriateness, educational requirements, cultural relevance, gender identification, other)

   Student is at an age and has telephone experience to manage phone conversation. Culturally, student needs to be cognizant of time of day and respectful of other person while carrying on conversation.

E. Acceptable Criteria for Completed Activity

   The purpose of the conversation is accomplished and the phone is placed back as initially found.

F. Activity Demands

   1. Objects and Their Properties

   a. Tools/Equipment (nonexpendable), Cost, and Source

      Telephone, $10.00, Wal-Mart
      Desk and chair, $70.00, Wal-Mart
      Address book, $3.00, Wal-Mart

   b. Materials/Supplies (expendable), Cost, and Source

      Access to phone lines, $20.00, Ameritech
      Cost of the call, $1.00, AT&T

FORM 3
ACTIVITY ANALYSIS FOR EXPECTED PERFORMANCE (CONTINUED)

2. Space Demands
   The activity requires sitting in a chair behind a desk in a quiet room at a comfortable temperature.

3. Social Demands
   The student should be aware of telephone etiquette when on the phone (e.g., to listen attentively, respond courteously, and be aware of the other person's role expectations).

Section 2: Analyzing Performance Areas of Occupation

A. Activities of Daily Living (ADL)
   1. Bathing, Showering

   2. Bowel and Bladder Management

   3. Dressing

   4. Eating

   5. Feeding

   6. Functional Mobility

   7. Personal Device Care

   8. Personal Hygiene and Grooming

   9. Sexual Activity

   10. Sleep/Rest

   11. Toilet Hygiene

B. Instrumental Activities of Daily Living (IADL)
   1. Care of Others

   2. Care of Pets

   3. Child Rearing

   4. Communication Device Use
      The phone call is used to convey information to another person.

FORM 3
ACTIVITY ANALYSIS FOR EXPECTED PERFORMANCE (CONTINUED)

    5. Community Mobility

    6. Financial Management

    7. Health Management and Maintenance

    8. Home Establishment and Management

    9. Meal Preparation and Cleanup

    10. Safety Procedures and Emergency Response

    11. Shopping

C. Education
    1. Formal Educational Participation

    2. Exploration of Informal Personal Educational Needs or Interests

    3. Informal Personal Education Preparation

D. Work
    1. Employment Interest and Pursuits

    2. Employment Seeking and Acquisition

    3. Job Performance

    4. Retirement Preparation and Adjustment

    5. Volunteer Exploration

    6. Volunteer Participation

E. Play
    1. Play Exploration

    2. Play Participation

F. Leisure
    1. Leisure Exploration

    2. Leisure Participation

FORM 3

ACTIVITY ANALYSIS FOR EXPECTED PERFORMANCE (CONTINUED)

G. Social Participation

    1. Community

    2. Family

    3. Peer, Friend
       Conversation with friend provides social outlet.

Section 3: Analyzing Performance Skills and Client Factors

Part I. Performance Skills

A. Motor Skills

    1. Posture (stabilizes, aligns, positions)
       I can maintain my balance while making the call in a sitting position; I can sit up straight in the chair while my feet remain on the floor throughout the phone call conversation.

    2. Mobility (walks, reaches, bends)
       Some large muscle movement in trunk, shoulder, and elbow for reaching motion is required.

    3. Coordination (coordinates, manipulates, flows)
       This is needed for me to turn pages in address book, lift receiver, and dial the numbers.

    4. Strength and Effort (moves, transports, lifts, calibrates, grips)
       Muscles allow arms and hands to move in a smooth way to complete the task.

    5. Energy (endures, paces)
       Sufficient tolerance to maintain length of time needed to hold phone and carry on a conversation, approximately 10 minutes.

B. Process Skills

    1. Energy (paces, attends)
       I'm alert enough to find the number in the address book and complete task of making the phone call. I know who and where I am so that a phone call can be made and I'm aware of the time of day and whether or not it is an appropriate time to make the call. I can recognize the task as one I have done before and with which I am familiar, as well as the voice of the person whom I'm calling. Adequate attention is needed to complete the call.

    2. Knowledge (chooses, uses, handles, heeds, inquires)
       I recognize the need to make a phone call to my friend, plan what I will say, note that I could email her or just wait, but decide to make the call, proceed with the call, and follow-up the conversation with the outcome upon which we decided.

FORM 3

ACTIVITY ANALYSIS FOR EXPECTED PERFORMANCE (CONTINUED)

3. Temporal Organization (initiates, continues, sequences, terminates)

   I am capable of and knowledgeable enough to sit at the desk, open the address book, and dial the number to begin the task of conversation with my friend. I am capable of ending the conversation in a timely manner. I can recall the purpose and procedure of making a call (e.g., the sequence of steps needed to complete the activity). I can perform all the steps necessary to make the call in the correct order.

4. Organizing Space and Objects (searches/locates, gathers, organizes, restores, navigates)

   I know to use an alphabetical order of names in the address book to find the correct name and number. I have encoded the concept of "making a phone call" and am able to organize incoming and outgoing information so as to convey my thoughts during the conversation.

5. Adaptation (notices/responds, accommodates, adjusts, benefits)

   I am able to respond to my friend's comments and accommodate to what she is saying, adjust my actions and words accordingly, and see the benefits of listening to her and making a collaborative decision about the time to meet.

C. Communication/Interaction Skills

1. Physicality (contacts, gazes, gestures, maneuvers, orients, postures)

   I make physical contact with the phone and can maneuver the theater schedule and address book as needed and orient myself to the information contained there.

2. Information Exchange (articulates, asserts, asks, engages, expresses, modulates, shares, speaks, sustains)

   I interact with my friend using verbal skills and active listening.

3. Relations (collaborates, conforms, focuses, relates, respects)

   I am able to collaborate with my friend and focus upon our decision, at the same time respecting her needs.

Part II. Client Factors

A. Body Function Categories

1. Mental Functions (affective, cognitive, perceptual)

   a. Global (consciousness, orientation, sleep, temperament and personality, energy and drive)

   I'm conscious of what I'm doing and oriented in all spheres of person, place, time, self, and others. I'm open to what my friend has to say and emotionally stable to handle this activity. I'm motivated to make the call and value my friendship for many reasons, but one is that we share the same interests.

   b. Specific (attention, memory, perceptual thought, higher-level cognition, language, calculation, motor planning, psychomotor, emotional, experience of self and time)

   I use all of these body functions to make the phone call (e.g., by attending to the activity for the length of time required to complete the task, making a decision, using the English language clearly, manipulating the phone and address book, staying calm as we talk, and aware of myself and the time of day).

2. Sensory Functions and Pain

   a. Seeing

   Scanning the environment, focusing on the phone, and reading the phone number.

FORM 3
ACTIVITY ANALYSIS FOR EXPECTED PERFORMANCE (CONTINUED)

b. Hearing/Vestibular

Listening to the friend converse and hearing one's self on the phone; I'm able to sit and keep my balance while using the phone.

c. Other (taste, smell, proprioception, touch, discrimination)

Proprioception is in place as I know where my body is in relationship to the desk and can feel the phone in my hand and can place it to my ear accurately. I touch the phone and can discriminate the receiver from the phone itself.

d. Pain

3. Neuromusculoskeletal and Movement-Related Functions

a. Joints and Bones (mobility, stability)

My joints allow me to maintain stability in a sitting position.

b. Muscle (power, tone, endurance)

I have sufficient strength to overcome gravity to hold the receiver to my ear and push the buttons to dial. Endurance is sufficient for entirety of activity.

c. Movement (motor reflex, reactions, voluntary, involuntary, gait)

Reflexes and reactions are intact to allow for voluntary movement.

d. Cardiovascular, Hematological, Immunological, and Respiratory

All these functions are operating within a normal range, allowing me to engage in this activity

e. Voice and Speech

These functions are actively engaged in this activity.

f. Digestive, Metabolic, and Endocrine

g. Genitourinary and Reproductive

h. Skin, Hair, and Nails

B. Body Structure Categories

1. Nervous System

These structures are intact and allow the functions described above to occur (i.e., voluntary movement).

2. Eye, Ear, and Related Structures

These structures are in place so that I may see and hear.

FORM 3
ACTIVITY ANALYSIS FOR EXPECTED PERFORMANCE (CONTINUED)

3. Voice and Speech
   These structures are in place so that I may talk clearly.

4. Cardiovascular, Immunological, and Respiratory
   These structures are in place so that I may engage in this activity of minimum energy.

5. Digestive

6. Genitourinary and Reproductive

7. Movement
   Allows for handling the objects and facilitates control so that my body responds to the activity demands.

8. Skin and Related Structures
   These structures are intact which then allows for touch, proprioception, and discrimination.

Section 4: Analyzing Performance Patterns and Contexts

Part I. Performance Patterns

A. Habits
   Useful in that it supports performance in daily life and contributes to life satisfaction.

B. Routines
   Making a phone call is an activity that has an established sequence.

C. Roles
   The role of friend and being connected.

Part II. Performance Contexts

A. Cultural
   The custom of making a phone call and meeting the behavior standards of such an activity are part of my environmental context.

B. Physical
   All the necessary nonhuman objects are present for me to conduct a phone conversation (e.g., desk, chair, phone, and address book).

C. Social
   The phone call serves as an available social outlet with my friend.

D. Personal
   I am a 25-year-old female student in college and able to manage such tasks as making a phone call.

FORM 3
ACTIVITY ANALYSIS FOR EXPECTED PERFORMANCE (CONTINUED)

E. Spiritual

Relating with a friend via a phone call is meaningful to me.

F. Temporal

I'm a young adult making a call in the evening during the school year.

G. Virtual

Making a phone call occurs by means of airways and an absence of physical contact.

NOTES

NOTES

NOTES

NOTES

Module III

Therapeutic Utilization of Activity

Unit 5

Activity Gradation and Adaptation

---

*Thus, the unique contribution of
occupational therapy is to maximize
the fit between what it is the individual wants
and needs to do and his or her capability to do it.*
(Christiansen & Baum, 1997, p. 40)

OBJECTIVES

Upon completion of this unit, the student will be able to:

* Define the terms *grading* and *adapting* as applied in occupational therapy intervention.
* Explain how grading or adapting activities can contribute to improving the client's performance.
* Give examples of a graded activity in each of the occupational performance areas.
* Give examples of adaptations in each of the occupational performance areas.
* Recognize specialty areas in service delivery related to grading and adapting activities.

With a thorough understanding of how to perform an activity, the student can begin to see ways in which the activity can be graded or adapted to meet specific client needs. Like analysis, there is no one way to grade or adapt activities. Both gradation and adaptation are used in the process of intervention to help a client change performance. The practitioner determines the intrinsic values within an activity through analysis and then may grade or adapt the activity to develop its potential value to a specific client (Trombly & Scott, 1977, p. 243). In this unit,

several approaches to grading and adapting activities will be shown.

"An occupational therapy practitioner grades or adapts a chosen activity for an individual to promote successful performance or elicit a particular response" (American Occupational Therapy Association [AOTA], 1993). For the purposes of this unit, grading will refer to changing the complexity of what is to be performed, and adapting will refer to modifying or substituting objects used in performing the activity.

GRADING

Grading activities are a part of daily life. Making a list of errands to do and checking them off as they are completed is a graded activity. Separating laundry into piles of dark- and light-colored clothes before placing them in the washing machine is another example. As the AOTA (1993) states:

> Grading activities challenge the patient's ability by progressively changing the process, tools, materials, or environment of a given activity to gradually increase or decrease performance demands. These incremental modifications are made in response to the individual's dynamic changes and provide opportunities for gradual development of skill and related therapeutic benefits.

Grading means to arrange or position in a scale of size, quality, or intensity. Grading can be compared to measuring how much of a specific task is performed. Most students experience "being graded" in school, in other words, how they measure up against a given standard. Grading involves setting a goal and then backing off to see how to complete it: the number of steps to be taken, the amount of time to be given each one, and the details required to perform them. In one sense, it is reversing the analysis of an activity. Performing the activity is the goal. The challenge is how the client will do the activity given specific strengths and limitations. The method used to reach that goal must be chosen by the therapist using professional experience and expertise to determine the appropriate means. Grading the activity is comparable to setting the stage for the client to succeed in performing it.

Some common examples of grading include:

* Breaking a lengthy activity into smaller units with given endpoints instead of tackling the entire job, such as reading one chapter of a weekly reading assignment each evening instead of trying to read all seven chapters in one sitting.

* Organizing items logically and in location according to priority use instead of having them in the general work area, such as placing writing utensils and paper on the desk on the dominant hand side.

* Changing the amount of energy needed by using lighter weight materials or tools to complete a project, such as working with softwoods (pine or poplar) instead of hardwoods in making a bookcase or using a power saw instead of a handsaw for cutting the wood.

* Increasing or decreasing the number of repetitions of an activity, such as walking a longer distance to improve endurance or doing less keyboard work to rest wrist extensors.

Another way of looking at grading is comparing the process to normal growth and development. As a toddler, it is normal to play with a telephone (real or replica) such as turning the dial or pushing buttons, holding the receiver, talking to an imaginary friend, and placing the telephone back in the cradle. As a child grows, the mechanical and proper use of a telephone takes on importance, including skills such as obtaining correct numbers, understanding the significance of these numbers, and listening as well as replying. Later, additional skills are added: to look up specific numbers by alphabetical order, to make and receive calls, respond courteously, limit phone conversations in time or subject, handle phone options such as call forwarding, and perform long distance or credit card calls. A toddler would not be expected to perform the activity of making a phone call on the same level as an adult. By grading the activity to what is appropriate to the individual's ability, the occupational therapy practitioner provides the setting, opportunity, and means for the individual to adapt and master the task.

For example, telephoning a beauty parlor to make an appointment is the purposeful activity chosen for a client experiencing mild confusion and problem-solving skills following a seizure. The therapist may grade the activity on a continuum from one extreme to the other based on the client's needs and progress as follows:

* All items assembled in one area for client use, gradually changing to the client locating and retrieving all items needed to perform activity.

* No time constraint placed on client to complete activity, gradually changing to a set amount of time in which to perform activity.

* Working without distraction in a quiet setting, gradually changing to working with background noise and frequent interruptions.

* Providing verbal cueing and a written sequence of steps, gradually changing to self-initiated activity.

* Role modeling the phone call, gradually changing to spontaneous independent performance.

Activity grading is used by the therapist to help a client improve performance level. Most activities involve overlapping use of multiple skills. In the above example of making a phone call, an activity analysis provides information that performance skills, performance patterns, context, activity demands, and client factors are all involved when performing this activity. Through gradual changes of the context, the client is provided the means for gradual improvement in occupational performance. "As a general rule, an activity should be graded up when the patient is able to accomplish the task and further progress is desired, or graded down when the patient is having difficulty with performance" (Levine & Brayley, 1991, p. 610).

Consider a graded exercise and activity program in a cardiac rehabilitation unit of a hospital. The first intervention session may involve passive range of motion to all extremities of the client and teaching proper breathing techniques. The client may be allowed to perform oral hygiene and feed self with the bed elevated at a 45-degree angle and with arms supported but is dependent on nursing for bathing and dressing. By the fourth session, the client may have progressed to performing active range of motion to all extremities with the bed in a 45-degree angle. The client may now be able to wash the front of the torso and use a bedside commode. By session eight, the client may be standing with 1- to 2-pound weights to perform range of motion exercises, bathe in a tub with assistance getting in and out, and begin independent dressing activities. The gradual increase in occupational performance can be well-documented and illustrates the use of grading.

Knowing the client's occupational history is an important resource for determining how to grade the activity. The individual's anxieties, interest level, and expectations regarding therapy help the practitioner determine where and how to focus on improving performance. In the above example, the activity of making a phone call to set up an appointment may range from being the infrequent task of a homemaker to the major job component of an executive assistant. The significance of performing specific components of this activity within a variety of activities versus performing this one activity successfully as part of the person's occupational needs is an important distinction to be made.

Another aspect of grading is looking at where occupational therapy intervention should begin. There are many types of standardized forms to "grade" the client's ability to function during an evaluation. Observing clients perform a functional task such as oral hygiene, feeding, dressing, or homemaking can pinpoint problems in attention, memory, initiation, safety and judgment, problem solving, visual tracking, body awareness, and/or motor planning. Through grading the client's performance, the practitioner identifies more precisely the specific disability. The intervention can begin at a point where the client successfully performs with subsequent sessions gradually increasing the demands on the client's occupational performance.

Every activity used in occupational therapy intervention should be gradable. With that prerequisite, every activity used has the potential for documenting the client's progress.

ADAPTATION

A background in the historical and conceptual use of the term *adaptation* in occupational therapy is beyond the scope of this book but is an important part of the student's education. A list of references is given at the end of this unit as a starting point for learning more. In one sense, the real goal of all occupational therapy is to facilitate the client's adaptive responses to promote health and well-being.

What is an adaptation? Simply put, something that makes doing some activity easier. Technically, an adaptation is a change in structure, function, or form that provides a better adjustment to the environment in which people live. For the purposes of this textbook, the term *adaptation* is being used as defined in the statement below:

> *Therapeutic adaptations refer to the design and/or restructuring of the physical environment to assist self-care, work and play/leisure performance. This includes selecting, obtaining, fitting and fabricating equipment, and instructing the client, family and/or staff in proper use and care of equipment. It also includes minor repair and modification for correct fit, position, or use.* (AOTA, 1979)

Adaptations surround us daily. As humans, we are constantly looking for ways to perform activities competently, effectively, and efficiently. Some common examples of adaptations are:

* Applying Velcro to serve as a fastener on the flap of a purse.
* Color coding files of information for quick retrieval.
* Recording foreign language phrases on a cassette to play/pause/repeat as needed.
* Marking the grain of the fabric with a safety pin to lay out a dress pattern.
* Wearing a Walkman to weed out unpleasant stimuli while working.
* Putting different textured surfaces onto individual keys to aid in finding the correct one.

Adaptation may require changing the tool or technique used to perform an activity. The therapist must judge whether or not to use a device to substitute for a specific performance component designed to function in place of the client's ability. Using a stationary cutting board to substitute for bilateral function in slicing vegetables or installing a grab bar in a bathroom to facilitate transfers are examples of adaptations.

Adaptations do not change the outcome of an activity, but the means of accomplishing the activity is purposefully altered to make it within reach of the client's ability. Looking up a phone number and dialing it may be a difficult task for the client experiencing hemiparesis, loss of memory from a head injury, or severe depression. Adaptations may include setting up a Rolodex to replace a phone book, learning to use a redial feature on a phone console, or plugging a headset into the receiver instead of handling the traditional one.

In some instances, the therapist may decide not to adapt the activity used in intervention. The client may be working to reach the same level of function before disability occurred, including doing the activity as it was "normally" performed prior to dysfunction. For example, a woman suffering from a stroke may benefit from using a plate guard while eating but be motivated to learn how to perform without it. The client may also resist or deny the need to have adaptations until the need is clearly demonstrated. For example, a person experiencing a double below-knee amputation may feel learning to wear prosthetics is discouraging and a bother until the desire to be independent in a public restroom provides the meaningful incentive for using them. The client may also have a preference to perform activities in a specific way despite the timeliness or expenditure of physical energy involved. The purpose and meaning attached to the way in which the activity is accomplished may be more important than making the task easier. For example, a man with multiple sclerosis may choose to use leg braces rather than a wheelchair to walk down the aisle at his daughter's wedding.

The therapist must know when to subordinate personal preferences to the client's desires, yet not jeopardize the welfare and safety of the client. Again, the context in which the client performs is an important component of knowing when an adaptation is needed and what is an appropriate one to use.

Occupational therapy practitioners are increasingly involved in delivering services in specialty areas of practice. Two of these are mentioned here because of their specific use of skills in adapting and grading activities. Ergonomics is a field of study using applied science to specifically adapt equipment and the surrounding work environment to maximize human productivity. Adapting working conditions to suit the worker includes the physical space, lighting, and sensory input, as well as tools and equipment.

Assistive technology is formally defined as "any item, piece of equipment, or product system, whether acquired commercially or off the shelf, modified, or customized, that is used to increase, maintain, or improve functional capability of individuals with disabilities" (Public Law 100-407, Technology-Related Assistance for Individuals with Disabilities Act of 1988). The use and development of technology or applied science has exploded in the past half century to affect people around the world in a myriad of ways. In all its varied shapes and forms, from basic devices such as long-handled reachers, to complex environmental control units, to general information technologies such as the Internet, assistive technology is within the scope of occupational therapy service delivery when applied to enhance an individual's performance. Technology can be an important tool to the practitioner when used appropriately to enhance an individual's occupational performance. Like prosthetics and orthotics, assistive technology is one of the categories of therapeutic adaptations.

The rapid pace with which changes and new developments are taking place in both ergonomics and assistive technology has created a demand for personnel with the proper qualifications to fill this need. Occupational therapists are well-suited to work in both of these fields because of their skill in adapting activities or the setting to match the individual's needs.

Three further points should be mentioned regarding grading and adaptation. First, it is important not to contrive inappropriate activities as a means of grading or adapting them to improve client performance—for example, having the client roll putty into pea-size balls to simulate eating them with a fork rather than dining with actual food and utensils in the cafeteria, or fastening a weight to a hanger to improve upper extremity strength and endurance rather than hanging a variety of garments of different weights. The activity should be meaningful as well as purposeful while matching goals of intervention. Whenever possible, substituting a simulated situation for the actual one in which the client will perform should be avoided. Realistic gradations rather than artificial ones should be provided as needed.

Second, the practitioner often must choose between fabricating an adaptation using clinic time and materials or buying a commercial product to do the same job. It may be more cost-effective to purchase a similar product and modify it to fit when received. On the other hand, a manufactured item may not be available or not have the capability of being customized for the individual and require the therapist to pursue other solutions. Similarly, in some instances it may be more efficient to have the client perform a commercially produced activity than to devise one to facilitate the desired response. Liability of the product used or the practitioner's own occupational readiness to perform certain physical modalities are other considerations. Again, knowledge, experience, and the individual client's response to the activity will enter into the decision of how the therapist will proceed with intervention.

Third, the practitioner must personally be able to grade and adapt professional performance. In other words, the therapist grades and adapts not only activities used in intervention, but also personal behavior to meet the client's needs. The therapist must adjust and "fit" modalities given multiple variables: the client's health status, time restraints, resources available, the acceptable practice standards, physician approval, and other therapy requirements to name a few. In a sense, the practitioner is the master role model of demonstrating adaptive behaviors and facilitating the adaptive response in the client's occupational performance.

DISCUSSION QUESTIONS

1. How have you changed in your ability to perform successfully in school since kindergarten? High school? College? How has "grading" influenced this ability?

2. What are some common adaptations you use in your own life? In what way do they make the activity easier to perform?

3. When you are ill, in what ways do you grade the activities you are able to perform?

4. Why are occupational therapy practitioners well-qualified to contribute in the fields of ergonomics and assistive technology?

REFERENCES

American Occupational Therapy Association. (1979). *Uniform terminology for reporting occupational therapy services.* Rockville, MD: Author.

American Occupational Therapy Association. (1993). Position paper: Purposeful activity. *American Journal of Occupational Therapy, 47,* 1081-1082.

Christiansen, C., & Baum, C. (1997). *Occupational therapy: Enabling function and well-being* (2nd ed.). Thorofare, NJ: SLACK Incorporated.

Levine, R. E., & Brayley, C. R. (1991). Occupation as a therapeutic medium: A contextual approach to performance interaction. In C. Christiansen & C. Baum (Eds.), *Occupational therapy: Overcoming human performance deficits* (pp. 591-631). Thorofare, NJ: SLACK Incorporated.

Public Law 100-407, Technology-Related Assistance for Individuals with Disabilities Act of 1988.

Trombly, C. A., & Scott, A. D. (1977). *Occupational therapy for physical dysfunction.* Baltimore, MD: Williams & Wilkins.

NOTES

NOTES

NOTES

NOTES

Unit 6

Activity Analysis for Therapeutic Intervention

OBJECTIVES

Upon completion of this unit, the student will be able to:

* Describe the therapeutic qualities of the activity.
* Identify possible gradation and modification strategies for the activity.
* Begin to formulate intervention outcomes for specific population-based groups.

Form 4 takes the student one step beyond activity analysis for expected performance. The intent is to have the student begin to think like a therapist. The potential for the activity to be purposeful and meaningful for intervention is explored. Here is where consideration of the activity as a therapeutic modality is addressed. To assist the student in translating the performance areas, skills, client factors, patterns, and contexts of the activity into a therapeutic mode of thought, this form is divided into three sections. Each section requires the student to think more intensely about the client's deficits and occupational performance in comparison to the expected activity performance.

SECTION 1:
ACTIVITY DESCRIPTION

The student provides a brief description of the activity being analyzed for therapeutic value and identifies the major steps in performing the activity. If this was com-

pleted in the learning phase, it need not be repeated now. However, as the student becomes more competent in this thought process, this section should be completed if the first form was not done. This will be especially true as new activities are added to the student's repertoire.

SECTION 2:
THERAPEUTIC QUALITIES

In this section, characteristics of the activity that have therapeutic potential are identified in terms of energy and activity patterns elicited by its performance. For example, when brushing one's teeth, a minimal work energy pattern is typically used as demonstrated through the body functions and structures of the cardiopulmonary system of the person. Students may want to refer to endurance data collected in the form of metabolic requirements of activities that are computed using metabolic equivalent units (METs). One MET represents the amount of energy it takes to rest while sitting in a semi-reclining position; accordingly, brushing one's teeth would equal 2 METs (Dutton, 1995, pp. 38-40). In turn, performance patterns characteristic of the activity may be exhibited (e.g., brushing teeth is characterized by methodical and repetitive actions and is considered a useful habit with an established sequence).

SECTION 3: THERAPEUTIC APPLICATION

This section allows the student to consider for whom and in what way engaging in the activity can enhance occupational performance. At this point, the student now applies the concepts of gradation and adaptation learned in Unit 5. Particular attention is given to ways in which the activity can be modified to a client's needs as well as how preventative measures may be implemented to facilitate optimal occupational performance. Finally, the student is asked to consider how the activity may play a part in the balance of the performance areas to enhance the health of the client.

Objective

Upon completion of Form 4, Activity Analysis for Therapeutic Intervention, the student will be able to address the therapeutic implications of any given activity.

Directions

* ✳ Describe activity demands and performance patterns, including energy patterns.
* ✳ Formulate possible intervention outcomes that could be derived from engaging in the activity.
* ✳ Explain gradation and adaptation possibilities.

* ✳ Specify therapeutic modifications that may be made to the activity with the client and/or to the environment to achieve identified goals.

Before completing this form, the student should review *Uniform Terminology* (AOTA, 1979) for definitions of terms used in the therapeutic modifications portion.

See the example of making a telephone call illustrated in Form 4.

DISCUSSION QUESTIONS

1. What have you learned about therapeutic implications that is most interesting to you? Most challenging?
2. What do you see as the next step in learning more about activity analysis?

REFERENCES

American Occupational Therapy Association. (1979). *Uniform terminology for reporting occupational therapy services.* Rockville, MD: Author.

Dutton, R. (1995). *Clinical reasoning in physical disabilities.* Baltimore, MD: Williams & Wilkins.

Moyers, PA. (1999). Guide to occupational therapy practice. American Journal of Occupational Therapy, 53(3): 247-322.

FORM 4
ACTIVITY ANALYSIS FOR THERAPEUTIC INTERVENTION

Student: Example _____ Date: _____

Activity: Making a telephone call _____

Course: _____

Section 1: Activity Description

A. Provide a Brief Description of Activity.

The student will prepare to make a telephone call, dial the number, convey a message to a friend, and close the conversation.

B. Identify Major Steps.
1. *Sit in chair comfortably.*
2. *Find phone number in address book accurately.*
3. *Pick up receiver carefully.*
4. *Listen for dial tone attentively.*
5. *Press phone number correctly.*
6. *Wait for an answer patiently.*
7. *Talk to person clearly.*
8. *Conclude conversation courteously.*
9. *Put receiver down firmly.*

Section 2: Therapeutic Qualities

A. Energy Patterns—Describe the required energy level in terms of light, moderate, or heavy work patterns and provide an explanation for the level specified. Consider the client factors of the cardiovascular and respiratory systems as well as muscle endurance.

Minimal work pattern needed to complete this task: MET level 1.8 to 2. The person needs to focus and organize self while preparing for task and to complete task. Cognitive awareness and required physical actions to perform the task demand some mental and physical exertion, but typically this is considered a sedentary activity.

B. Activity Patterns—Indicate the patterns of the activity expected for successful completion of the activity.
1. Structural/Methodical/Orderly

   Steps of activity provide structure and order to perform task (e.g., have address book available to find number, pick up receiver, and use phone to dial number).

2. Repetitive

3. Expressive/Creative/Projective

   Verbal expression is utilized during the conversation to exchange thoughts and ideas.

4. Tactile
   a. Contact With Others (e.g., hands-on, stand by assist)

      This task does not require contact with others.

FORM 4
ACTIVITY ANALYSIS FOR THERAPEUTIC INTERVENTION (CONTINUED)

    b. Materials (e.g., pliable, sensual)

Hands and fingers are touching the cover and pages of address book; hand, fingers, face, and ear are on receiver; fingers touch the dial; and body sits on chair. Materials are mostly of a solid surface except for pages of book.

    c. Equipment (e.g., size, manageability, shape)

Telephone is of the right size and shape for effectively managing the call; desk and chair are appropriate for task.

C. Performance Patterns.

  1. Habits

Useful in that it supports performance in daily life.

  2. Routines

Making a phone call involves an established sequence.

  3. Roles

I'm a friend and student.

Section 3: Therapeutic Application

A. Population—Discuss for whom and in what way increased occupational performance can be derived from the use of this activity. Consider the motor, process, and communication/interaction skills. Identify any contraindications.

This activity falls in the performance area of IADL, particularly communication device use and in social participation with a friend/peer. In the motor realm, it promotes posture and alignment of body to desk and materials; reaching for objects; coordination and manipulation of hand use; strength and effort to use objects; and sustaining effort long enough to make the phone call. In the process skill area, knowledge to seek and participate in a phone conversation and organizing space and objects can be challenged; temporal organization in being able to initiate, continue, sequence, and terminate the activity is also expected. Predominantly, it focuses on the communication/interaction skill area to reinforce physicality, information exchange, and maintain relations. No apparent contraindications, unless social behaviors are severely dysfunctional or there is a possibility the phone could be used abusively.

Population-based groups in which this activity could have applicability are deficits in fine motor coordination/dexterity and grasp as seen with muscle weakness or paralysis; process deficits in sequencing, attention to activity, problem-solving; and psychosocial problems of social conduct and interpersonal skills.

B. Gradation—Describe ways to grade this activity in terms of:

  1. Activity Sequence, Duration, and/or the Activity Procedures

The activity sequence could be graded from supervision by a practitioner to independent performance of client (e.g., instructions could be written or in picture format, the task could be broken into smaller parts for easier manageability, or client could be asked to initiate and implement task on own).

Duration of call could be shortened or lengthened, depending on client's capabilities or purpose of call.

Activity procedure could be altered by using different types of communication (e.g., email or cellular phone). It could be done with a friend or stranger. Purpose of call could vary from utilitarian as a request for information to more social and friendly conversation.

  2. Working Position of the Individual

The client could be asked to stand by a wall phone, sit in another type of chair, or make call from a bed and/or asked to retrieve materials for task, depending upon the endurance of the client.

FORM 4
ACTIVITY ANALYSIS FOR THERAPEUTIC INTERVENTION (CONTINUED)

3. Tools
   a. Position

   The phone and address book can be placed in various planes depending upon the needs of the client for easier or more challenging access.

   b. Size

   Various types of phones are available that could "match" the needs of the client (e.g., a cellular phone, larger numbers, dial numbers, or touch tone).

   c. Shape

   The same for size of phone could apply here as well.

   d. Weight

   Again, depending on the type of phone, weight may vary.

   e. Texture

   This is an area that probably does not lend itself to gradation as much as the others.

4. Materials
   a. Position

   b. Size

   c. Shape

   d. Weight

   e. Texture

5. Nature/Degree of Interpersonal Contact

   The nature of the interpersonal contact is indirect in that there is no face-to-face interaction; however, it may still vary in objective or subjective information being exchanged (e.g., a call could be made to a stranger, such as a request for pizza delivery or for a business transaction, or it could be made to a friend or relative with whom the client may feel close).

6. Extent of Tactile, Verbal, or Visual Cues Used by Practitioner During Activity

   The practitioner could vary the amount of assistance from maximum cues and "hands-on" facilitation initially and gradually lessen the physical and cognitive supervision needed for the client to complete the task independently.

FORM 4
ACTIVITY ANALYSIS FOR THERAPEUTIC INTERVENTION (CONTINUED)

7. The Teaching-Learning Environment

The environment could be adjusted to meet the needs of the client in a variety of ways (e.g., the room itself could be quiet with little distractions or the client could be asked to make the call at a busy traffic intersection on a public pay phone; space and placement of tools could change, from a large desk to a kitchen phone by a small counter).

C. Therapeutic Modifications—Indicate ways in which this activity may be changed to increase occupational performance. State your reasoning. Write n/a if not applicable. Definitions for the following terms can be found in Appendix B, *Uniform Terminology for Reporting Occupational Therapy Service, First Edition,* "Therapeutic Adaptations" and *The Guide to Occupational Therapy Practice* (AOTA, 1999).

1. Therapeutic Adaptations

   a. Orthotic Devices

     If needed, an orthotic device or splint could be created to help the client grasp the receiver.

   b. Prosthetic Devices

     In this case, training with the prosthesis may be necessary for the client to learn to manipulate the pages of a book, receiver, and dialing or punching numbers.

   c. Assistive Technology and Adaptive Devices

     (1) Architectural Modification

       Chair and desk should be ergonomically correct for maintaining posture or workstation could be built into an area if space is a consideration.

     (2) Environmental Modification

       The room may need to be carpeted to soften sound or temperature controlled, again, depending on the needs of the client.

     (3) Tool and Equipment Modification (low-tech [e.g., reacher] or hi-tech [e.g., computer control devices])

       Enlarged numbers on phone for those who are visually impaired, a TDD device for those hearing impaired, or speaker phone for someone who has difficulty with arm motion and hand/finger manipulation are just some possibilities.

     (4) Wheelchair Modification

       A lap tray can be used instead of a desk, or the wheelchair may require desk arms to fit under the workstation. Footrests may need to swing away, or if needed, be adjusted comfortably for foot support.

2. Prevention

   a. Energy Conservation

     (1) Energy-Saving Procedures

       Address book should be at the desk ready for use to avoid having to locate it. The phone number could be in the phone memory so it is accessible by the push of one button instead of ten.

FORM 4
ACTIVITY ANALYSIS FOR THERAPEUTIC INTERVENTION (CONTINUED)

(2) Activity Restriction

Client may be asked to restrict self from making too many calls, which may make him or her feel fatigued.

(3) Work Simplification

As mentioned earlier, using phone memory and having all materials at hand will make the activity simpler for the client.

(4) Time Management

In terms of social conduct or endurance, for example, the client may need to be reminded to make calls at only appropriate times or limit calls.

(5) Environmental Organization

Items on desk should be organized in such a way that the client can reach them easily. Desk, chair, and phone should be easily accessible for normal use as well as for emergency situations.

b. Joint Protection/Body Mechanics

(1) Using Proper Body Mechanics

Especially for reaching items, client may need to be reminded of proper movement patterns; and for sitting, a chair with good trunk, arm, and leg support is needed. Elbows could rest on desk to keep arms from tiring.

(2) Avoiding Static/Deforming Postures

The client may need to be reminded to maintain good body posture and limit use of the phone, providing rest periods as needed.

(3) Avoiding Excessive Weight-Bearing

This shouldn't be a problem if the client is sitting while making a call. If standing, proper body mechanics should be emphasized.

c. Positioning

Depending upon the placement of the phone, positioning could take on many forms. Regardless if the client is standing or sitting, good body mechanics and ergonomically correct body posture are essential.

d. Balance of Performance Areas to Facilitate Health and Well-Being

(1) Enhancement of Occupational Performance Areas

The areas of communication device use and social participation will be enhanced by the client through this task performance.

(2) Satisfaction of Client and/or Caregiver

In this case, the client will feel pleased that he has been able to complete a call and converse with a friend.

(3) Quality of Life

Feeling good about "doing" a task by one's self and being in touch with a positive support system contributes to one's well-being.

Notes

NOTES

NOTES

NOTES

Unit 7

The Client-Activity Intervention Plan

OBJECTIVES

Upon completion of this unit, the student will be able to:

* Identify the areas of occupational deficit as found in the client's occupational profile.
* Prioritize and develop long- and short-term goals that will address these deficits.
* Select, describe, prepare, and implement a purposeful activity that will enhance occupational performance.
* Document the occupational outcome.

Form 5, The Client-Activity Intervention Plan (CAIP) provides a method of synthesis for all the information developed through the use of the previous four forms. The CAIP develops the relationship between the client's present deficits in occupational performance and the purposeful activity selected as the strategy for intervention. The CAIP is a step-by-step outline for a single treatment intervention. It begins with the referral and occupational history, outlines the practitioner's role in the preparation for and administration of an intervention sequence, and documents the intervention outcomes. This approach is illustrated in the Occupational Therapy Process (Moyers, 1999), which describes the occupational therapy protocol for treating a client. The Occupational Therapy Process begins with the referral of the client to occupational therapy services; progresses through the evaluation phase, the development of the intervention plan, the intervention itself, and subsequent reevaluation; and concludes with either discharge or further follow-up.

The CAIP addresses the second stage of the *Occupational Therapy Practice Framework* and outlines the overall development of the intervention plan. Here, the practitioner and the client together identify realistic and meaningful goals that address the deficits in the client's occupational performance. For the student working through an intervention sequence, the CAIP organizes the learning that has culminated through the use of the Activity Awareness, Action Identification, and Activity Analysis forms. The student now moves into the areas of occupation that are meaningful to the client and appropriate to the development of the client's occupational competence. The CAIP provides a five-step organizational design that demonstrates the development of long- and short-term intervention goals, the choice of the purposeful activity to be used as an intervention strategy, the practitioner's preparation sequence, the intervention sequence itself, and the recording of the documented outcomes that are guided by the use of the *Occupational Therapy Practice Framework* (AOTA, 2002).

GOALS OF THERAPY

By combining professional expertise and clinical reasoning with the information gained from the client's referral, evaluation measures, and from other professionals, the occupational therapy practitioner develops the long- and short-term goals of therapy. These goals denote intervention outcomes and project the way that carefully selected activities will facilitate improvement in the client's occupational performance. The goals and the activities must demonstrate a therapeutic and meaningful relationship with each other and to the client. Each goal and its accompanying purposeful activities must clearly demonstrate the progress the client will be expected to make during the intervention process.

Long-Term Goals

A long-term goal indicates the expected outcome of the intervention and focuses on improving the client's occupational performance. In clearly defining each long-term goal, the practitioner projects the client's occupational performance at the time of discharge. Long-term goals frequently include a specific period of time or number of treatments. However, current health care guidelines may dictate that intervention will address only some of the client's immediate needs. Intervention may be further constrained by payment for a limited number of treatments. In today's market, the practitioner must continually employ creative and resourceful clinical reasoning skills to effectively address the client's most immediate and realistic goals for performance.

Short-Term Goals

A long-term goal is supported by short-term goals that are activity centered and are a sequence of one or more units of accomplishment that must be completed to reach each long-term goal. Short-term goals are described as a series of building blocks of activity that are purposefully selected, sequenced, and graded to lead to the occupational performance defined by the long-term goal.

A CASE STUDY

The following example demonstrates how one long-term goal requires the completion of seven short-term goals.

Occupational Profile

Bobby Jones is a 9-year-old boy who frequently misses the school bus. If his parents have left for work by the time he misses the bus, he is absent for the day. Bobby is capable of meeting the school bus but he is easily distracted. To successfully participate in his occupational role as a student (Performance in Areas of Occupation, Instrumental Activities of Daily Living), he needs to independently use school bus transportation to get to school (Community Mobility).

Occupational Therapy Intervention

After interviewing Bobby and his parents, the occupational therapy practitioner develops long- and short-term goals for intervention and will coach Bobby and his parents on the best way for Bobby to get to the bus on time.

Long-Term Goal

At discharge, the client will demonstrate independence in routinely using school bus transportation 4 out of 5 mornings per week.

Short-Term Goals

To demonstrate independence in using school bus transportation, the client will do the following:
* Dress appropriately for weather conditions.
* Carry a backpack containing his lunch and all required school materials.
* Self-monitor the time he must leave home using his new self-selected watch with a built-in timer.
* Arrive at the bus stop 5 minutes before the scheduled stop.
* Board the bus in a sociably accepted manner.
* Quickly find a vacant seat.
* Remain seated until the bus driver discharges the students at school.

Both long- and short-term goals have to be observable (i.e., student routinely uses the bus successfully), measurable (i.e., student arrives at school on time and in a socially acceptable manner at least 4 out of 5 days), and expressed in behavioral terms (i.e., the client will...).

Progress Note Example

Following 2 weeks of occupational therapy intervention, the client successfully demonstrates his independence in using the school bus to get to school on time and in a prepared manner. His parents and teacher have noted his independence.

According to the *Occupational Therapy Practice Framework*, the goals respond to the Performance Area of Occupation (Instrumental Activities of Daily Living-Community Mobility) and require Performance Skills (Motor and Process Skills), Performance Patterns (Habits, Roles, and Routine) and Context (Physical and Temporal), and Client Factors (Global Mental Functions).

Because accountability, occupational performance, and cost containment are prime criteria for the reimbursement of occupational therapy services, the use of occupation as intervention must be justifiable. When writing either long or short-term goals, the practitioner must clearly demonstrate that these goals are occupational in intent and are within the guidelines of occupational therapy practice. As in the Activity Analysis Process, domain and process terminology can be used to document the client's level of performance.

Clinical Reasoning

The student now begins to realize that each short-term goal is made up of one or more purposeful activities that are used to fulfill the requirements of that goal. Consider the series of activities that are required to complete short-term goal #3:

* The client will don his new watch upon awakening in the morning.
* The client will set his timer to indicate the time he must leave the house.
* The client will frequently check the time while dressing and eating breakfast.
* The client will understand the amount of time required to cover the distance between his home and the bus stop.
* When his timer rings, the client will independently leave home in time to meet the bus.

These five steps define the bus meeting activity required to meet short-term goal #3. The student may also realize that each of the steps listed above could become a goal with its own series of steps imbedded in an action sequence.

CLIENT-ACTIVITY INTERVENTION PLAN: AN OVERVIEW

The Occupational Profile

As in practice, all intervention begins with a referral of a client who will benefit from occupational therapy services. The CAIP form begins with a brief outline of the client's occupational history and profile. In this text, the occupational profile information used in preparing the CAIP form (Form 5) will be more specific than is generally found in practice. This approach is used to narrow the range of goals the student has to consider at this point in the learning process. However, in today's practice, a practitioner may find it necessary to screen the available client population, decide who could benefit from occupational therapy intervention and in what way, and then approach a physician with a request for a referral if necessary.

Intervention Goals

Long- and short-term goals are developed from the information found in the client's occupational profile. While the need for several long-term goals may be evident, the beginning student should think about the client's most immediate goal. In our case example, it was tempting to list his occupation as student only. However, at the time of intervention, he was clearly in the role of student. His goals needed to focus on his community

mobility so he could fulfill his role of student. With the meaningful long-term goal firmly in mind, the student can then begin the clinical reasoning process required to analyze the client data and develop the short-term goals that support that one long-term goal. As the student progresses academically and professionally, the amount of client information readily available through other professional resources will increase. The student will then be required to discern and prioritize increased opportunities for occupational therapy intervention.

Intervention Activity Description

This section requires a brief description of the activity and how it will be used therapeutically. This description is similar to the activity description completed earlier in Section 1 (Activity Summary) of the Activity Analysis form.

Intervention Activity Preparation

Prior to actual contact with the client, the practitioner needs to set aside a period of time to plan and prepare for the therapy session. After reviewing the client's areas of deficit and determining the purposeful activity that will be used to address a specific goal, the practitioner develops a preparation plan by considering some or all of the following questions:

* Have I analyzed all the ramifications of the selected purposeful activity so that I can competently employ it in a therapeutic manner? Am I ready to make adaptations as necessary?
* Do I have all the required equipment, materials, and supplies? Will I need to place an order? If so, what is my time line between ordering, receiving, and the intervention?
* Where is the most appropriate place to treat this client and what context factors must I consider?
* I must make an appointment with the client. Are there others I should contact as well?
* Will I do my preparation in my office, the clinic, or another site?
* How long will my preparation take?
* Can I do my preparations independently or will I need assistance? If so, who?
* Do I need to negotiate transportation for my equipment and myself or will the client come to a clinical area?
* What personal safety precautions should I observe as I make my preparations?

For professional credibility, the session should be completed without the distracting frustration that results from insufficient knowledge, incomplete preparation, or poor organization on the part of professional personnel. While unforeseen circumstances may sometimes disrupt a treatment session, the habit of thorough preparation is an asset to both the practitioner and the client. Preparation time may be included in the treatment charge for occupational therapy services. Documentation time and consultation with other practitioners or caregivers may also be included.

Intervention Activity Implementation

The client, the practitioner, and all materials and equipment must be in place at the stated time. Depending on the nature of the activity being used, additional personnel may be needed to assist or observe during the intervention period. Co-treating practitioners, client caregivers, technicians, vendors, aides, and students are potential personnel. The setting has to be large enough to accommodate all personnel and necessary equipment. Lighting, room temperature, a calming or stimulating atmosphere, privacy issues, and client's accessibility to the room and its furnishings are some of the important environmental factors to be considered. These criteria are suggested in the context area of the domain section of *Occupational Therapy Practice Framework*.

During the intervention period, the occupational therapy practitioner needs to be attuned to the client's physical, cognitive, and psychological condition. If any part of the activity appears to compromise the client's status or safety, the practitioner may need to shorten the session or grade and adapt the activity before continuing.

Intervention Activity Sequence

Using purposeful activity as an agent for change in promoting occupational performance is unique to occupational therapy. Clear and concise documentation of the methods used and the occupational performance that results are necessary for the client's records. Therefore, the documentation of the activity sequence used by the practitioner must be more than a listing of a series of steps resembling ingredients in a cookbook. In the Action Identification form, the student used the Do-What-How format to document the action observed in one's self or by another. In the CAIP, the student expands the Do-What-How concept by adding additional elements: "with what" (performance skills and performance patterns) and "under what circumstances" (context). The student is already familiar with the Performance Skills, Patterns, and the Performance Context as they were used in the Activity Analysis Form. Return to the example of activities used by the young client learning to use school bus transportation and identify statements that indicate this Do-What-How, with what and under what circumstances approach. Are the short-term goals fulfilled?

The therapist documents the major steps of the activity and indicates the therapeutic value. The major steps—not the incidental ones—performed by the client reveal the therapeutic value. If the activity contains more than a few steps that are not of therapeutic value or the practitioner must do most of an activity for the client, then a more relevant activity should be chosen. Generally, the therapeutic steps of an activity can be documented in 10 steps or less. It is important to clearly identify the role of the practitioner throughout the intervention. The documentation should demonstrate how the presence and expertise of an occupational therapy practitioner is required to successfully complete the intervention and should be stated in behavioral terms.

Example: Selecting and activating the appropriate numbers on a push-button phone.

Given verbal instruction and hand-over-hand guidance by the therapist, the client will accurately select and activate the required phone number.

Intervention Documentation: Domain and Process

The final section of the CAIP is the documentation of the therapeutic outcomes resulting from the specific intervention. This documentation should reflect the agenda from the referral and demonstrate how the purposeful activity selected as the agent for intervention has generated a change in the client's occupational performance. The *Occupational Therapy Practice Framework* suggests the domain, in which the therapeutic intervention was conceived, and the process, which denotes the criteria of implementation. Consider again the young client working on using school bus transportation.

Domain

Our young client was working in the occupational areas of instrumental activities with emphasis on community mobility. He received intervention in his performance skills (motor and process), performance patterns (habits and routines), contexts (physical, social, and temporal), and client factors (global mental functions).

Process

The intervention approach for this client was to establish and maintain a routine to assure that he could independently and appropriately use public school bus transportation. Occupation-based activity was the type of intervention. The outcomes included occupational performance, client satisfaction, and role competence.

The student is cautioned to use only those terms that actually identify the therapeutic outcomes. Frequently, students using the CAIP for the first time tend to revert back to the Activity Analysis format, which requires a response to all items required to perform an activity. In the Activity Analysis documentation, the student must focus on all the areas of the domain that the successful completion of the activity places on the client. In the CAIP, the documentation focuses only on the areas of the domain and process that demonstrate the attainment of the occupational goals that were outlined in the occupational profile. Justification for the use of each item is not required with this form.

REFERENCES

American Occupational Therapy Association. (2002). Occupational therapy practice framework: Domain and process. *American Journal of Occupational Therapy, 56*, 609-639.

Moyers, P. (1999). The guide to occupational therapy practice [special issue]. *American Journal of Occupational Therapy, 53*(3), 247-322.

Webster's New World College Dictionary (3rd ed.). (1997). New York, NY: Simon & Schuster, Inc.

Form 5
Client-Activity Intervention Plan

Student: Example   Date:
Action: Making a phone call
Course:

1. Client Occupational Profile and Referral

   A. Client Occupational Profile

   The client is a 67-year-old male who is progressively loosing his sight due to complications of diabetes. He is now 2 years postretirement from his position as a senior clergyman in a large local church. Upon retirement and, because of his diminishing vision, he requested permission to initiate a phone ministry to the homebound members of his church. His duties include weekly phone calls to approximately 40 elderly or disabled members to provide social contact and church information or arrange assistance when necessary. He worked from a small office in his church. He was successful in keeping in touch with members who came to depend on his weekly call. When his failing vision reduced his community mobility, the church members began looking for a way for him to continue his ministry from his home. At the time of the referral, the client could no longer drive his car or safely walk the three blocks from his home to his office at the church. Public transportation was inadequate. He has a large, sunny study in the first floor of his home, which he now shares with a large parrot and an old Siamese cat. His wife has been deceased for 3 years. He has been referred to occupational therapy for evaluation and assistance in converting part of his study into a home office. He needs to use the phone independently and be able to record information because he no longer has the assistance of the church secretary.

   B. Referral

   Evaluate and intervene to develop independence in using the telephone and to seek ways to record received information in a manner compatible with his diminishing vision.

2. Intervention Goals

   A. Long-Term Goal (First Priority)

   The priority goal for the client is to be able to make phone calls and record usable information independently.

   B. Short-Term Goal (Support)

   1. The client and practitioner will select a telephone and a recording device that best fits his needs.
   2. The client and the practitioner will develop a workstation in his home study.
   3. The client will independently call one of his parishioners from his new telephone.

3. Intervention Activity Description

   The client will experiment with several types of telephones equipped with assistive technological features to find one that best fit his needs. The practitioner will research the market and provide several examples of existing models.

4. Intervention Activity Preparation

   A. Review Goals and Describe Practitioner's Role

   In view of the goals stated above, the practitioner will survey professional technology catalogs to determine the types of phones currently on the market. The practitioner will also confer with the assistive technology staff of the large state rehabilitation center in a neighboring city for further information. With the permission of the technology staff, the practitioner will arrange to borrow three different styles of telephones for 1 week to determine the client's independent use before a permanent purchase is made. The practitioner will carefully learn to use all of the features of each phone before meeting with the client as well as seek resources for funding the purchase of the telephone. The practitioner will arrange to meet the client at his home 3 weeks from today.

FORM 5
CLIENT-ACTIVITY INTERVENTION PLAN (CONTINUED)

B. Personnel Required to do the Preparation
One practitioner

C. Required Preparation Time
Approximately 3 weeks

D. Required Place and Space
The practitioner will work from the clinic office.

E. Materials
Office supplies

F. Equipment
Desk, chair, telephone, phone book, and catalogs

G. Safety Precautions for Personnel
None required

5. Intervention Activity Implementation
   A. Personnel
   Client and practitioner

   B. Setting and Location
   Client's home study

   C. Space Required
   Easy access to and around the client's workstation (desk)

   D. Environment
   Quiet and undisturbed: remove parrot (noise factor) and cat (curiosity)
   Lighting of the workstation and room temperature should be at comfortable levels.

   E. Materials
   Calendar (large print), note pad with wide lines, and pen or pencil

   F. Equipment: Assistive Devices or Adaptations Included
   Equipment will include clear desktop space, two chairs, three assistive telephones with recording features, convenient wall jack for phone, and a rolling card file with names and phone numbers in large print.

   G. Required Intervention Time
   1.5 hours. In addition to setting up the equipment and experimenting with each phone, the client and practitioner need time to thoroughly consider the features of each and have ample opportunity to try them as often as necessary.

   H. Safety Precautions for Client
   There should be an unobstructed pathway from the doorway of the study to the chair at the desk. The desk should be free of clutter. The three phones should be within easy reach to facilitate easy comparison.

FORM 5
CLIENT-ACTIVITY INTERVENTION PLAN (CONTINUED)

6. Intervention Activity Sequence (10 action steps or less)

   A. *The client will seat himself at his desk.*

   B. *The therapist will place one phone on the desk within his working range.*

   C. *After determining the phone to be in working order, the therapist will verbally and tactilely describe its working features.*

   D. *The client will follow the practitioner's directions in using each feature.*

   E. *The practitioner will observe the ergonomic aspects of the client's use of the phone and make recommendations for increasing his work comfort and efficiency.*

   F. *This sequence will be repeated for the other two phones.*

   G. *The client and the practitioner will evaluate the positive and negative features of each phone.*

   H. *The client will select the phone that offers him the most independence.*

   I. *The client will select a name and number from his card file and successfully make a phone call.*

   K. *The client will record that person's response for future use.*

7. Documentation

   A. Domain

      1. The Areas of Occupation: Instrumental Activities of Daily Living (communication device use) and Work (Job Performance)

      2. Performance Skills: Process Skills (adaptation), Communication Skills (information exchange)

      3. Performance Patterns (routines and roles)

      4. Activity Demands (objects and their properties, space demands)

      5. Client Factors (sensory function-seeing and related functions)

   B. Process

      1. The type of Occupational Therapy Intervention used with this client was the consultation process. The practitioner provided expertise, examples, and research information that assisted the client in selecting communication equipment that met his goal of making a phone call independently.

      2. The types of outcomes include improved occupational performance, client satisfaction, and role competence.

NOTES

NOTES

NOTES

Module 4

The Versatility of Activity

Throughout the first three modules, the use of activity as the instrument for change in the client's occupational performance has been demonstrated in a variety of ways. Activity performance has been brought to the surface from the subconscious level and cognitively acknowledged. The required steps of an activity have been graded, adapted, added to, reduced, and rearranged. Activity is viewed as a universal requirement for a meaningful quality of life and serves as the building block of occupation.

In the second and third modules, the simple activity of making a phone call was utilized as a teaching tool to develop the progressive understanding and use of the five forms presented in the text. The phone call activity was first called into consciousness and observed through Forms 1 and 2. It was reduced to its elements in Form 3 and then reassembled with all its therapeutic implications in Form 4. In Form 5, it was used to demonstrate a plan of intervention in an occupational setting for an adult client.

In Unit 8, a simple activity is again being used sequentially through all five forms. These examples are used to further illustrate the versatility of activity as occupational therapy intervention. In the first four forms, the activity is examined as before. This time the fifth form, the application portion of the process, demonstrates the use of a goal-directed activity in a group therapy setting. In this example, the elements of a cookie-baking activity are organized by the practitioner to facilitate an increase in the socialization skills of a small group of young school-age children, each with a different disability.

In Unit 9, the student is provided with the instructions for using the Web site containing all five forms used in this text. This allows the student to have easy access to all or part of each of the forms as class assignments require; the forms can be used easily and often. This makes activity analysis and its application to occupation a portable educational tool that can be used in the classroom, during fieldwork, and eventually in the work place. Use of the Web site as an effective reporting tool can further demonstrate the range of occupational therapy services to the public.

Unit 8

A Review of the Process

FORM 1
ACTIVITY AWARENESS FORM

Student: Example _____   Date: _____

Activity: Making cookies from a recipe _____

Course: _____

Directions: Reflecting on the activity just performed, complete the following sentences with the first words that come to mind.

1. During this activity I was thinking about...
   The times my mom and I would make cookies as a kid.

2. While doing this activity I felt...
   I should do this more often. It's a lot of fun.

3. In doing this activity, the parts of my body I remember using were...
   My fingers and hands, my tongue to taste, and my nose to smell.

4. To do this activity I need to...
   Pay attention so I don't add the wrong ingredient or leave the pans in the oven too long.

5. When I do this activity again I will...
   Set it up at a counter with chairs so we can all sit down to work. Also I would make a double recipe.

6. From doing this activity I became aware of...
   How much I enjoy baking, especially the smells, and eating homemade items.

FORM 2
ACTION IDENTIFICATION FORM

<u>Student: Example</u>   <u>Date:</u>
<u>Activity: Making cookies from a recipe</u>
<u>Course:</u>

Directions: Select an activity, and using the Do-What-How style, list the major actions in sequence in 10 steps or less required for you to perform this activity. Repeat the exercise after observing someone else perform the same activity.

Observation of Self

1. Assemble the recipe ingredients appropriately.
2. Measure out the ingredients and mix them thoroughly.
3. Preheat the oven correctly.
4. Grease the cookie sheets sparingly.
5. Spoon and drop the dough on the sheet spacing leniently.
6. Put filled sheets in the oven and set the timer accurately.
7. Wait for the cookies to bake patiently.
8. Remove sheets and put cookies on wax paper carefully.
9. Wash dishes and counter completely.
10. Eat cookies eagerly.

Observation of Another

1. Read the directions thoughtfully.
2. Find and lay out the ingredients and utensils thoroughly.
3. Preheat the oven and prepare the trays accurately.
4. Follow the recipe carefully.
5. Place the dough on the trays appropriately.
6. Put the trays in to bake and set the time correctly.
7. Set the dishes to soak efficiently.
8. Remove the cookies cautiously.
9. Clean the dishes and kitchen area completely.
10. Sit down and eat cookies contentedly.

FORM 3
ACTIVITY ANALYSIS FOR EXPECTED PERFORMANCE

Student: Example   Date:
Activity: Making cookies from a recipe
Course:

Section 1: Activity Summary

Directions: Respond to the following in list format.

A. Name and Brief Description of Activity

Making cookies from a recipe. The student will read the recipe directions for chocolate chip cookies, gather necessary tools and ingredients, prepare dough according to recipe directions, and bake the cookies.

B. Sequence of Major Steps (in 10 steps or less; specify time required to complete each step)

Read recipe directions	*2 min.*
Gather necessary ingredients and utensils (assuming they are already available in kitchen)	*5 min.*
Preset oven temperature	*30 sec.*
Measure and mix ingredients	*10 min.*
Place mixed dough on baking sheet	*5 min.*
Place baking sheet in the oven	*1 min.*
Set oven timer	*30 sec.*
Bake cookies until timer sounds; check for doneness	*15 min.*
Remove baking sheet from oven	*1 min.*
Remove cookies from baking sheet with spatula and place on cooling racks	*5 min.*

Total time = 45 minutes.

C. Precautions (review "Sequence of Major Steps")

When baking cookies, it is imperative that the student use an oven mitt upon placing the baking sheet in or when removing the sheet from the oven. An oven mitt must also be used while removing the cookies from a hot baking sheet with a spatula. Also, it is important that the student understands the proper safety procedures used when operating an oven and that quantities of ingredients or baking temperatures should not be altered.

D. Special Considerations (age appropriateness, educational requirements, cultural relevance gender identification, other)

To complete this activity, the student must be able to read, comprehend mathematical concepts such as fractions, and be capable of operating an oven. No set gender identification needs to be made. Culturally, the person would value and have an interest in cooking and preparing food for self or others. In many subgroups of society this task is highly looked upon and respected.

E. Acceptable Criteria for Completed Project

The finished product of this activity are cookies that are golden brown, edible and tasty, and of an appropriate size to be eaten by hand.

F. Activity Demands
   1. Objects and Their Properties
   a. Tools/Equipment (nonexpendable), Cost, and Source

   The tools and equipment needed for baking cookies can be purchased in the housewares department of a retail establishment. These items include the following:

FORM 3
ACTIVITY ANALYSIS FOR EXPECTED PERFORMANCE (CONTINUED)

Mixing bowl	*$3.00*
Mixing spoon	*$1.00*
Measuring cups	*$1.00*
Measuring spoons	*$1.50*
Baking sheet	*$3.00*
Cooling racks	*$3.00*
Spatula	*$1.00*
Oven mitt	*$3.00*

An oven with a built-in timer (on hand, no recent cost expended)
The total cost for nonexpendable tools and equipment is $16.50.

  b. Materials/Supplies (expendable), Cost, and Source

The ingredients necessary for making chocolate cookies can be purchased at a grocery store. Materials and supplies needed include the following:
Flour
Eggs
Granulated white sugar
Brown sugar
Salt
Butter
Chocolate chips
Nuts
Baking powder
Vanilla
Also, gas or electric energy is required to operate the oven
The total cost for expendable items is less than $10.00.

2. Space Demands

To perform this activity, it is necessary to have a kitchen facility with adequate counter space (approximately 5 ft.).

3. Social Demands

No interaction will take place with others, but student should be cognizant of cleaning the kitchen so others may use it when needed. It's possible that cookies are being made for a social function or as a gift.

Section 2: Analyzing Performance Areas of Occupation

A. Activities of Daily Living (ADL)
  1. Bathing, Showering

  2. Bowel and Bladder Management

  3. Dressing

  4. Eating
    Cookies will be eaten following preparation and baking.

FORM 3
ACTIVITY ANALYSIS FOR EXPECTED PERFORMANCE (CONTINUED)

5. Feeding

6. Functional Mobility
Moving about the kitchen to retrieve tools and ingredients for cooking and baking purposes is considered functional mobility.

7. Personal Device Care

8. Personal Hygiene and Grooming
Washing hands prior to making cookies.

9. Sexual Activity

10. Sleep/Rest

11. Toilet Hygiene

B. Instrumental Activities of Daily Living (IADL)

1. Care of Others

2. Care of Pets

3. Child Rearing

4. Communication Device Use

5. Community Mobility

6. Financial Management

7. Health Management and Maintenance
Cooking and baking could be considered maintenance of health, such as nutrition.

8. Home Establishment and Management
It is possible that when purchasing ingredients, the student will need to be aware of the cost of items. If there is a limited budget, generic or store brands could serve as an alternative to more expensive name brands. To perform a baking activity, the student will want to ensure that all equipment (e.g. oven, refrigerator, water faucets) are clean and in working order.

9. Meal Preparation and Cleanup
The student will prepare cookies, open and close containers, use an oven, and manipulate kitchen utensils. Cleanup will take place as well.

10. Safety Procedures and Emergency Response
Safety is part of this activity when using kitchen utensils and the oven.

FORM 3
ACTIVITY ANALYSIS FOR EXPECTED PERFORMANCE (CONTINUED)

11. Shopping

    The student may need to shop for ingredients, but for this particular activity all ingredients were available in the kitchen.

C. Education

   1. Formal Educational Participation

   2. Exploration of Informal Personal Educational Needs or Interests

   3. Informal Personal Education Preparation

D. Work

   1. Employment Interest and Pursuits

   2. Employment Seeking and Acquisition

   3. Job Performance

   4. Retirement Preparation and adjustment

   5. Volunteer Exploration

   6. Volunteer Participation

E. Play

   1. Play Exploration

   2. Play Participation

F. Leisure

   1. Leisure Exploration

   2. Leisure Participation

      Baking cookies may serve as a leisure skill for the student, providing an enjoyable activity to the person.

G. Social Participation

   1. Community

   2. Family

   3. Peer, Friend

      Giving cookies to another may be considered a way of interacting and sharing others. Also, cookies could be prepared in a group setting.

FORM 3
ACTIVITY ANALYSIS FOR EXPECTED PERFORMANCE (CONTINUED)

Section 3: Analyzing Performance Skills and Client Factors

Part I. Performance Skills

A. Motor Skills

1. Posture (stabilizes, aligns, positions)

   It is necessary for me to maintain a standing posture while mixing the cookie dough at the counter and use proper posture while placing items in and removing items from the oven. In order to maintain good body mechanics, such as when bending at knees instead of waist when placing cookies in oven, I need to keep trunk in good alignment with other parts of body.

2. Mobility (walks, reaches, bends)

   I need to be able to walk about the kitchen and reach for items on counter or in a cabinet; bending is required when placing in and taking out the cookies from the oven.

3. Coordination (coordinates, manipulates, flows)

   Large muscle groups at shoulder, trunk, and hips are under active control in order for me to move around the kitchen, mix the dough, carry the pans and stand upright. Throughout this task, fine coordination of hand and fingers are in high demand as I measure ingredients, manipulate utensils, and place cookie dough on the pans.

4. Strength and Effort (moves, transports, lifts, calibrates, grips)

   Fair plus to good strength is needed to lift ingredients, mix the dough, maintain an erect posture, and transport pans to oven. I need enough stamina to begin and complete the task in the time allotted. Grip is needed to hold small utensils, like a spatula.

5. Energy (endures, paces)

   Sufficient tolerance to maintain length of time needed to complete the activity of making cookies, approximately 30 to 60 minutes.

B. Process Skills

1. Energy (paces, attends)

   Alertness is essential when working in the kitchen handling ingredients for predetermined quantities and being cognizant of safety concerns. I know who I am, the time of day, and where I am in order to complete this activity, e.g., I'm an adult who is making cookies for a friend; it's morning and I have sufficient time to complete the activity before going to class and am in the appropriate room of the house, the kitchen, in order to complete the activity effectively. I am familiar with all tools and ingredients needed for activity completion and able to focus on the activity for the allotted time necessary.

2. Knowledge (chooses, uses, handles, heeds, inquires)

   I have the ability to seek and use task-related knowledge. For example, I taste and look at the dough to determine if the ingredients are fresh and in proper proportion to one another. I also may need to determine when substitutions of ingredients are needed or how to correct errors with baking times and oven temperatures. Acquiring new ideas about baking may take place, e.g., the cookies are burned and I realize the oven temperature is off or baking time needs adjustment, so that next time that is prevented from happening; or, I realize that I can make substitutions in the recipe and the cookies taste even better!

FORM 3
ACTIVITY ANALYSIS FOR EXPECTED PERFORMANCE (CONTINUED)

3. Temporal Organization (initiates, continues, sequences, terminates)

It is apparent to me when I can start this activity, as I know the time, feel motivated, and have the needed ingredients to begin. I know that there is only a certain amount of time to complete the activity and am aware that when the cookies are done baking and I've cleaned up after myself, it can be considered finished. I need to be able to place information and actions in order to complete the activity so that cookies are properly prepared, e.g. I need to grease the cookie pans before placing the cookies by spoonful onto cookie pan for baking.

4. Organizing Space and Objects (searches/locates, gathers, organizes, restores, navigates)

This skill area is essential for me to have in making cookies as I must be able to: locate and gather the tools and ingredients in a logical manner, organize them in the workspace so they are close at hand, restore the kitchen to its original condition, e.g. put away the flour and sugar in sealed containers, and navigate myself around the kitchen safely, avoiding any spills or knocking over of ingredients.

5. Adaptation (notices/responds, accommodates, adjusts, benefits)

If I smell smoke from the oven, I must respond accordingly to prevent burning the cookies. It's possible that if an ingredient is not available, I can accommodate and find a substitute; being able to adjust to any changes in the environment is needed as well, e.g., turning on the vent to air out the kitchen.

C. Communication/Interaction Skills

1. Physicality (contacts, gazes, gestures, maneuvers, orients, postures)

I'm doing this activity by myself, so this skill is not expected of me.

2. Information Exchange (articulates, asserts, asks, engages, expresses, modulates, shares, speaks, sustains)

Same as #1.

3. Relations (collaborates, conforms, focuses, relates, respects)

Same as #1.

Part II. Client Factors

A. Body function Categories

1. Mental Functions (affective, cognitive, perceptual)

a. Global (consciousness, orientation, sleep, temperament and personality, energy and drive)

I need to be conscious and oriented to name, place, time, and self when working in the kitchen handling ingredients for predetermined quantities and being cognizant of safety. I value my friendship and wish to share cookies with my friend as a token and gift of our friendship. Baking is an interest of mine which enjoy doing.

b. Specific (attention, memory, perceptual, thought, higher-level cognition, language, calculation, motor planning, psychomotor, emotional, experience of self and time)

I need to sustain attention to complete the task; I remember baking cookies and can generalize to the present activity. All of my perceptual functions are in place including motor planning and interpretation of sensory stimuli, e.g. touch, vision, and olfactory. Problem-solving and time management are being challenged by this activity. I feel good about myself while doing this activity.

2. Sensory Functions and Pain

a. Seeing

Vision to read recipe, ingredient labels, timer, and assess cookies for doneness and hearing for timer are called upon while doing this activity.

FORM 3
ACTIVITY ANALYSIS FOR EXPECTED PERFORMANCE (CONTINUED)

b. Hearing/Vestibular

I need to maintain my balance as I maneuver about the kitchen.

c. Other (taste, smell, proprioception, touch, discrimination)

As noted above, my senses are being challenged by the stimuli imparted from the engagement in a baking activity.

d. Pain

Only if I burn myself on the oven or baking pan!

3. Neuromusculosketetal and Movement-Related Functions

a. Joints and Bones (mobility, stability)

Physiologically, my joints and bones allow me to move about the kitchen efficiently.

b. Muscle (power, tone, endurance)

Sufficient muscle strength and endurance is needed to complete the activity.

c. Movement (motor reflex, reactions, voluntary, involuntary, gait)

Reflexes and reactions are intact allowing me to perform voluntary movement.

d. Cardiovascular, Hematological, Immunological, Respiratory

My cardiovascular and respiratory are functioning sufficiently so that I can engage in the activity without shortness of breath, few rest breaks, and no swelling of legs while standing.

e. Voice and Speech

Not needed in this activity, unless I find myself humming or singing a tune!

f. Digestive, Metabolic, Endocrine

Upon eating any cookies, I will digest them without problem.

g. Genitourinary and Reproductive

h. Skin, Hair, Nail

Only that my skin is in contact with the tools and work areas; in some instances, I may wish to pull my hair back.

B. Body Structure Categories

1. Nervous System

These structures are essential for me to engage in the activity.

2. Eye, Ear, and Related Structures

The eyes allow me to visualize the activity and the ear to hear the timer.

3. Voice and Speech

4. Cardiovascular, Immunological, Respiratory

These structures are essential in order to engage in any activity.

FORM 3
ACTIVITY ANALYSIS FOR EXPECTED PERFORMANCE (CONTINUED)

5. Digestive
   If I decide to eat any cookies, my digestive system needs to be in working order!

6. Genitourinary and Reproductive

7. Movement
   For me, this is essential while moving around and working in the kitchen

8. Skin and Related Structures
   These structures allow me to perceive and touch my environment accurately.

Section 4: Analyzing Performance Patterns and Contexts

Part I. Performance Patterns
A. Habits
   Useful in that this activity supports performance in daily life.

B. Routines
   Making cookies requires an established sequence.

C. Roles
   The role of homemaker and friend.

Part II. Performance Contexts
A. Cultural
   Baking cookies is a valued activity of my cultural group of peers and family, and one that is looked upon positively.

B. Physical
   The activity takes place in a kitchen so that I have access to the oven, sink, counter space, refrigerator, proper utensils, and ingredients.

C. Social
   I am working alone.

D. Personal
   I am a 24 year old female student.

E. Spiritual
   Making cookies to give as a gift and share with others is meaningful to me.

F. Temporal
   I'm a young adult and have designated this time to make cookies.

G. Virtual

Form 4
Activity Analysis for Therapeutic Intervention

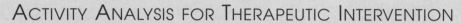

Student: Example   Date:
Activity: Making cookies from a recipe
Course:

Section 1: Activity Description

A. Provide a Brief Description of Activity.

The student will read the recipe directions for chocolate chip cookies, gather necessary tools and ingredients, prepare dough according to recipe directions, and bake cookies.

B. Identify Major Steps
1. *Read recipe directions.*
2. *Gather necessary ingredients and utensils.*
3. *Preset oven temperature.*
4. *Measure and mix ingredients.*
5. *Place mixed dough on baking sheet.*
6. *Place baking sheet in the oven.*
7. *Set oven timer.*
8. *Allow cookies to bake in oven.*
9. *Remove baking sheet from oven when timer sounds.*
10. *Remove cookies from baking sheet and place on cooling rack.*

Section 2: Therapeutic Qualities

A. Energy Patterns—Describe the required energy level in terms of light, moderate, or heavy work patterns and provide an explanation for the level specified. (Refer to description of MET levels in Unit 6). Consider the client factors of the cardiovascular and respiratory systems as well as muscle endurance.

A moderate work pattern is used to complete this activity. A MET level of 2.5 to 3.0 is used in this activity. The person needs to be sufficiently focused and organized to prepare and complete the cookie baking, as well as physically able to move about in the setting and to handle the utensils and equipment. Both cognitive and physical demands are placed upon the person but they are not physically and mentally exhausting.

B. Activity Patterns—Indicate the patterns of the activity expected for successful completion of the activity.
1. Structural/Methodical/Orderly

   Making cookies has all three characteristics, as the person must follow the steps listed in the recipe, be able to break an egg and know how to measure, and maintain some order to the process so ingredients are not used in error, and the kitchen is kept somewhat clean and neat.

2. Repetitive

   The steps of mixing the dough, dropping dough by spoonfuls onto cookie pan, and removing cookies one by one from the pan all have a repetitive pattern to them.

3. Expressive/Creative/Projective

   The person expresses his friendship and giving through the art of making cookies; one could easily be creative with substitution in the dough mix and with decorating cookies.

FORM 4

ACTIVITY ANALYSIS FOR THERAPEUTIC INTERVENTION (CONTINUED)

4. Tactile
   a. Contact With Others (e.g., hands-on, stand by assist)
   As this activity is being performed, there is no contact with others.

   b. Materials (e.g., pliable, sensual)
   While performing this activity, there is the feel of the dough, which is soft and pliable to the touch, or of other ingredients, which may be liquid or solid.

   c. Equipment (e.g., size, manageability, shape)
   While doing this activity, the person handles the utensils, oven, refrigerator, and counter top and typically, these tools and equipment are of the correct size and shape for managing most kitchen tasks.

C. Performance Patterns
   1. Habits
   Useful, as this activity supports performance in daily living.

   2. Routines
   Making cookies has an established sequence.

   3. Roles
   I am a friend and student who is capable of making cookies and sharing them with others.

Section 3: Therapeutic Application

A. Population—Discuss for whom and in what way increased occupational performance can be derived from the use of this activity. Consider the motor, process, and communication/interaction skills. Identify any contraindications.

This activity falls in the performance areas of activities of daily living, specifically eating and functional mobility; instrumental activities of daily living, including health management and maintenance, home establishment and management, meal preparation and clean up, safety procedures, and shopping; leisure participation; and possibly social participation with peer/friend if participating or sharing cookies with others. This kind of activity lends itself to almost all the performance skills; however, it specifically is useful with the following: motor—alignment of standing position while working at the kitchen counter, positioning body and arms to activity to cooking utensils, walking, reaching and bending in order to complete the cooking activity, and coordination of bilateral motor acts along with sufficient effort to complete activity; process—having the knowledge to use and handle tools as needed (e.g., with recipe measurements, sequencing, and organizing materials in the kitchen work space, and adapting to the cooking situation, in case an error is made and being able to adjust to the circumstances); communication/interaction—n/a as this is done as a solitary act.

Contraindications may be indicated for those who cognitively cannot grasp safety procedures or for those who may be self-destructive with utensils/tools. Also, any clients with a contagious illness may need to be excluded, and any diet restrictions, like diabetes, may need to be monitored.

Population-based groups in which this activity may have applicability are stroke and geriatric clients for training in an activity of daily living and homemaking or as an esteem builder for clients with psychosocial deficits. Anyone requiring standing tolerance and endurance would be appropriate. This activity can also be used for persons with brain injuries who need to practice activity planning and following directions. This activity has applicability to almost any age group from pre-school through adulthood as it can be adapted in a variety of ways to "fit" the needs of the client group. Its versatility is what makes it so appealing for many types of clinical and community settings.

FORM 4

ACTIVITY ANALYSIS FOR THERAPEUTIC INTERVENTION (CONTINUED)

B. Gradation—Describe ways to grade this activity in terms of:

1. Activity Sequence, Duration, and/or the Activity Procedures

   The sequence of the activity could be altered to match the needs of the client in a variety of ways (e.g., using a boxed cookie mix or even refrigerator cookie mix to lessen the steps). The amount of supervision could vary from hands-on to only stand-by assistance.

   Duration of activity could be shortened or broken into short periods of rest, if needed by the client, depending on the person's endurance, attention span, or capabilities.

   Activity procedure could be graded, as above, with different kinds of recipes presented to client; other possibilities are using an electric mixer instead of a spoon to mix, having all ingredients premeasured, or have the therapist place cookie pans in oven for safety concerns. To eliminate the hazard of oven use, cookies that can be baked in the microwave are a possibility.

2. Working Position of the Individual

   The client could sit at a table for preparing the dough, rather than standing. Sitting and standing could be alternated to provide rest breaks.

3. Tools
   a. Position

      The cooking utensils could be placed at different sites on the counter for easier or more challenging reach. However, the layout of the kitchen equipment will dictate accessibility.

   b. Size

      Bowl size could vary for easier handling.

   c. Shape

      Shape of handles of utensils may be varied for easier grasp.

   d. Weight

      Mixing bowls and spatula could be weighted for easier handling.

   e. Texture

      Possibly the feel of the tool handles may vary.

4. Materials
   a. Position

      Ingredients could be premeasured for easier access or the client may be asked to retrieve ingredients on his or her own.

   b. Size

      Larger or smaller amounts of cookie dough could be made depending on the purpose of the activity.

   c. Shape

Form 4

Activity Analysis for Therapeutic Intervention (continued)

    d. Weight

    e. Texture

    The nature of the dough could be altered to be more crunchy or smooth, depending on the recipe and desired taste.

5. Nature/Degree of Interpersonal Contact

    Interpersonal contact could be graded from a solitary act to a group activity. Supervision could vary from hands-on, guided, or stand-by depending on the needs of the client.

6. Extent of Tactile, Verbal, or Visual Cues Used by Practitioner During Activity

    The practitioner could vary the amount of assistance from maximum cuing and "hands-on" facilitation initially and gradually lessen the physical and cognitive supervision needed for the client to complete the task independently. Directions could be given verbally, by demonstration, by pictures, in large print, or a combination of these methods.

7. The Teaching-Learning Environment

    The environment of the kitchen setting could vary from a simulated kitchen in a clinic; a mock-up work area with table, chair, and utensils only; or an actual home visit. The area could be graded from distraction free to the typical noise of a clinic. Again, depending upon the needs of the client, the teaching-learning possibilities vary.

C. Therapeutic Modifications—Indicate ways in which this activity may be changed to increase occupational performance. State your reasoning. Write n/a if not applicable. Definitions for the following terms can be found in Appendix B, *Uniform Terminology for Reporting Occupational Therapy Services, First Edition,* "Therapeutic Adaptations" and *The Guide to Occupational Therapy Practice* (AOTA, 1999).

    1. Therapeutic Adaptations

        a. Orthotic Devices

        If needed, an orthotic device or splint could be created to help the client grasp the spatula.

        b. Prosthetic Devices

        Meal preparation provides a client who has an upper or lower extremity prosthesis to practice skills (e.g., for the upper extremity amputation, making cookies demands the person use the prosthesis with a variety of utensils, and for the lower extremity amputation, standing tolerance is facilitated).

        c. Assistive Technology and Adaptive Devices

            (1) Architectural Modification

            This is an area in which more or less modification could be done in the kitchen to facilitate or challenge the person, again depending upon the purpose of the activity and the needs of the client. For example, a workstation at wheelchair height could be built instead of using a counter top. Or, cabinets could have pull-out drawers and turn tables for easier access.

            (2) Environmental Modification

            Flooring, space, lighting, and temperature are considerations.

Form 4

Activity Analysis for Therapeutic Intervention (continued)

(3) Tool and Equipment Modification (low tech [e.g., reacher] and hi tech [e.g., computer control devices])

Several kinds of adaptations can be made to the tools and equipment (e.g., mixer stand, built-up handles, a cart to carry cookie pans to oven, a ledge on the counter top to prevent items from moving during preparation, a suction cup, or a coiled damp towel to hold the measuring cup or the mixing bowl).

(4) Wheelchair Modification

A wheelchair tray could be attached for easier handling of the utensils if a counter top is inaccessible. Leg rests that swing away and desk arms allow the person closer access to work station.

2. Prevention
    a. Energy Conservation
       (1) Energy-Saving Procedures

       Having all utensils and ingredients at hand lessens exertion. Sitting while mixing the dough, breaking the activity down into smaller steps, preparing the dough first and refrigerating it, then later completing baking are energy-saving options.

       (2) Activity Restriction

       As noted above, the activity can be broken down into smaller steps, rest breaks can be provided, and the activity can be divided into preparation and baking stages.

       (3) Work Simplification

       An electric mixer could be used to simplify the activity of mixing, or again the activity could be broken down into smaller steps. Assistance could be provided as needed.

       (4) Time Management

       To conserve time, the ingredients and supplies could be gathered at one time. Making cookies should be done at a time that allows for all steps to be completed, or plan ahead how best to divide the activity into stages, so one could be delayed without spoiling prepared dough.

       (5) Environmental Organization

       Supplies and ingredients could be gathered and placed together on the counter space before preparation is started. Working in a kitchen area that allows for easy access to supplies and ingredients needs to be considered.

    b. Joint Protection/Body Mechanics
       (1) Using Proper Body Mechanics

       During the performance of the activity, the client should use proper body mechanics such as bending from the knees instead of the waist, not overstretching to reach for items from cabinets, and if sitting at the workstation, have a chair with good trunk, leg, and foot support. A reacher may be indicated for some clients.

       (2) Avoiding Static/Deforming Postures

       Work surface height should be appropriate for standing or sitting while making cookies.

FORM 4

ACTIVITY ANALYSIS FOR THERAPEUTIC INTERVENTION (CONTINUED)

(3) Avoiding Excessive Weight-Bearing

The therapist should monitor this especially if client has limited standing tolerance or low endurance.

c. Positioning

The activity can be done in a sitting or standing position; either way, the practitioner should make sure that the client has good support and uses good body mechanics.

d. Balance of Performance Areas to Facilitate Health and Well-Being

(1) Enhancement of Occupational Performance Areas

The areas of meal preparation, functional mobility, and possibly leisure participation will be enhanced by performing this activity.

(2) Satisfaction of Client and/or Caregiver

The client will be happy with the completion of this activity and being able to share the cookies with a friend. Positive self-concept is a likely outcome.

(3) Quality of Life

Receiving satisfaction from completing such an activity as making cookies contributes to one's well-being, as it provides a sense of accomplishment and social connection in gift giving.

FORM 5
CLIENT-ACTIVITY INTERVENTION PLAN

Student: Example   Date:
Activity: Making cookies from a recipe
Course:

1. Client Occupational Profile and Referral
   A. Group Occupational Profile

   The occupational therapy practitioner assigned to School #27 is working weekly with a group of five third graders (clients) who have varying disabilities. Kent and Bruce have learning disabilities. Megan has mild Down syndrome. Peter has attention deficit disorder and Cynthia has juvenile rheumatoid arthritis and uses a power chair. She is frequently withdrawn and irritable. The therapist has been focusing on group-centered activities that will facilitate acceptable levels of social and communication skills within the group to help them increase their positive interaction with each other as well as their classroom peers.

   Initially, each child demanded excessive personal attention. Sharing and cooperation skills were weak. Their frustration level was high, their attention span was short, and they showed general inability to problem solve. Megan and Kent have limited communication skills, which sometimes leads to hitting or shouting. As of this date, the group has been together for 1 month. They have made some progress in using the phrases of "please, thank you, and please pass..." instead of grabbing from each other. They are now able to sit in a circle and pass items quietly from left to right. They are able to follow simple two-step directions without demonstrating frustration.

   B. Referral

   Evaluate and intervene to further develop each child's communication and social interaction skills.

2. Intervention Goals
   A. Long-Term Goal (First Priority)

   The priority long-term goal for each of these children is to be able to interact socially and cooperatively within their group setting within 2 months.

   B. Short-Term Goals (Support)

   1. The children will select a simple group activity that they would enjoy doing together.
   2. The children will agree to focus on their group interaction skills as they complete their activity.

3. Intervention Activity Description

   The Parent-Teacher Association of School #27 is sponsoring a bake sale next Tuesday and all the classes are invited to participate. The practitioner and the children discussed baking cookies together as their way to participate in the bake sale. The group voted to make chocolate chip cookies from a recipe and to use fresh ingredients.

4. Intervention Activity Preparation
   A. Review Goals and Describe Practitioner's Role

   In view of the goals for increased group interaction and cooperation, the occupational therapy practitioner will choose a chocolate chip cookie recipe and determine how each child can participate in the process of baking cookies. The practitioner will visit the school kitchen supervisor to request permission to use space in the kitchen for 1 hour and 15 minutes and to select a date for the activity. Together they will select the baking equipment the children will use. The practitioner will request the help of an aide from the kitchen staff to assist during the session. The practitioner will also request permission to walk the children through the kitchen the week before the activity to acquaint them with its sights and sounds and to meet the aide. When all the arrangements are in place, the practitioner will shop for the cookie ingredients and store them until they are needed.

FORM 5
CLIENT-ACTIVITY INTERVENTION PLAN (CONTINUED)

B. Personnel Required to do the Preparation
One practitioner

C. Required Preparation Time
Approximately 1.5 hours

D. Required Place and Space
School kitchen to evaluate working space and equipment
Grocery store to shop for the ingredients
Refrigerator space for ingredients

E. Materials
Shopping list
Sufficient funds for purchasing the ingredients

F. Equipment
Transportation to the grocery store

G. Safety Precautions for Personnel
Usual awareness while traveling and shopping

5. Intervention Activity Implementation
   A. Personnel
   Practitioner, the children, and one school aide

   B. Setting and Location
   The activity will take place in the school kitchen during the mid-afternoon period when the kitchen is not in use.

   C. Space Required
   Space is needed for two cafeteria tables and four chairs. Five children and two adults need to be able to move around the tables easily. The space surrounding the work area should be restricted so the children cannot wander away but can focus all their attention on participation in the table activity. Cynthia will need wheelchair space at the table.

   D. Environment
   The environment should be as calm as possible. This will be a challenge in a large, open kitchen with all the stainless steel workspace and appliances. Covering the children's workspace with clean bath towels will help dampen the noise and prevent utensils from sliding. The practitioner and the aide will use quiet voice tones as they direct the children. Since the children have already seen their work area, they should be less overwhelmed with its newness.

   E. Materials
   Chocolate chip cookie recipe, cookie ingredients, extra shortening for the cookie sheets, paper towels to wipe up spills and sticky fingers, cups and napkins, juice to enjoy with finished cookies, and a large plastic trash bag

   F. Equipment: Assistive Devices and Adaptations Included
   Small equipment includes a medium-size, nonbreakable mixing bowl; a small electric mixer; mixing spoons; measuring cups and measuring spoons; metal spatula; two cookie sheets; two cooling racks; a small basket for serving cookies; a large plastic container for storing the finished cookies; a timer; and bath towels to cover the tables. Two six-person tables and four chairs will be brought from the cafeteria. One will be the children's worktable and the other will hold the equipment and supplies. The kitchen oven is near the workspace.

FORM 5
CLIENT-ACTIVITY INTERVENTION PLAN (CONTINUED)

G. Required Intervention Time

One hour for the activity and 15 minutes for set up and clean up

H. Safety Precautions for Clients

Because all of the children have patterns of unpredictable behavior, they must be monitored closely to keep them on task. Cynthia will need help in handling large or heavy objects. Megan and Peter often throw things they cannot control. Kent and Bruce may not understand directions the first time. The practitioner and the aide must closely supervise the children so they use the materials and equipment carefully and effectively.

6. Intervention Activity Sequence (10 action steps or less)

A. While the practitioner is positioning the children around the worktable, the aide will measure each of the ingredients into a separate bowl small enough for each child to carry and place each bowl on the supply table. The mixing bowl and mixing spoon will be placed on the worktable.

B. The practitioner will read the name of an ingredient followed by a child's name, then direct or assist each child in going to the supply table to pick up the bowl containing the assigned ingredient and return to the table. The aide will assist the child in choosing the correct bowl if necessary.

C. When the children are seated, the mixing bowl will be passed from left to right and each child will add an ingredient to the bowl.

D. The mixing bowl will be passed a second time and each child will have a turn at mixing the contents with a mixing spoon. Both practitioner and the aide will assist as necessary. The aide will do the final mixing with a hand mixer.

E. As the bowl is passed again, each child will place a spoonful of cookie dough on a prepared cookie sheet. The practitioner may need to assist the placing of the dough with a spatula.

F. The aide will place the filled cookie sheets in the preheated oven. The timer will be set on the table where the children can watch it.

G. While the aide supervises the baking, the practitioner and the children will talk about the cookie baking process and how each child participated. The therapist will point out the positive aspects of their behavior as they worked together. The children will be encouraged to talk about their feelings and accomplishments. Each child will be encouraged to verbalize ways to improve their behaviors next time the group meets.

H. When the timer rings, the aide will remove the cookies from the oven and place them on cooling racks. Seven cookies will be placed in a small basket.

I. The children will pass the cookie basket around the circle from left to right. Each child will select one cookie and enjoy the treat. The children will share their cookies with the aide and therapist. Cups of juice and a napkin will be passed to each child.

J. Everyone will help clean up the work site and the cooled cookies will be placed in a covered plastic container ready to go to the bake sale. The practitioner and the children will thank the aide for helping them.

7. Documentation

A. Domain

The children's primary area of intervention is in the occupational performance area of social participation. While motor and process skills are evident, communication and interaction are the main focus in the performance skills. From the performance patterns, each child's role as a member of an interactive group was addressed. The intervention was centered in the physical, social, and personal context for each child.

B. Process

The occupational therapy approach to this intervention is the modification of each child's ineffective social behaviors and the establishment of acceptable interactive social skills. The intervention was an occupation-based activity (making cookies to enter into a school-based activity) that required social interaction and cooperation. The project was completed successfully through adequate occupational performance as demonstrated by client satisfaction (the children were pleased with their accomplishments) and role competence (each one felt he or she did his or her part).

NOTES

NOTES

NOTES

Unit 9

Utilizing Assistive Technology: The Forms Web Site

Your book has been provided with a colored insert (located inside the front cover) that contains your individual password to use the *Activity Analysis: Application to Occupation, Fifth Edition* Web site, located on the Internet at:

http://www.slackbooks.com/forms

Here you may download blank copies of the following forms free of charge:

* Activity Awareness (Form 1)
* Action Identification (Form 2)
* Activity Analysis for Expected Performance (Form 3)
* Activity Analysis for Therapeutic Intervention (Form 4)
* Client-Activity Intervention Plan (Form 5)

Please be sure to read the instructions that appear on the Web site carefully before proceeding to download them onto a disk or onto your computer's hard drive.

The five forms are for your personal use in the classroom or in your practice.

If you encounter any problems in downloading your *Activity Analysis: Application to Occupation, Fifth Edition* forms, please email SLACK Incorporated's Technical Support at Techsupport@slackinc.com or call 856-848-2186 Monday through Friday 9:00 am to 5:00 pm, Eastern Standard Time.

Epilogue

There is a story that carries remarkable impact for occupational therapy practitioners. Two fishermen were fly casting in a stream when they noticed with dismay a group of children floating down the river. Some of the children were struggling to remain above the water, others were floundering unsuccessfully, a few were managing to make it ashore unaided. The men abandoned their poles to help rescue the children, but more and more continued to come down the river. Suddenly, one of the fishermen rushed to the shore and started running upstream along the bank. The other called out to him not to leave because he could not manage to save the children alone. The departing fisherman yelled back, "Save those you can. I'm going to stop the person who's pushing them in" (West, 1973, p. 19). This story bears an analogy to the community and was originally given to introduce a range of issues facing health professionals. It also suggests some remarkable parallels to what the student has experienced in using this text. Analyzing what activity was needed in the situation dictated the occupational performance needs of both fishermen. The meaning and purpose of their occupation changed when a further aspect of the problem surfaced in the mind of one fisherman. The steps to make real intervention is revealed in the drastic decision to leave the other fisherman.

This handbook has been presented as a framework for thinking about activity in all its dimensions. Learning the process of activity analysis is a basic skill that all occupational therapy students must have before applying it toward an intervention model. The authors have offered the student a beginning level of knowledge in how activities can be used in intervention and relate to specific goals of a given client. "To use purposeful activity therapeutically, (a practitioner) analyzes the activity from several perspectives. ...all this information is considered together to assist... in synthesizing (i.e., adapting, grading, and combining) activities for therapeutic purposes for a particular

individual" (American Occupational Therapy Association, 1993). Purposeful activity is the medium of occupational therapy, and activity analysis serves as a baseline for understanding the importance of this concept.

Until recently, the use of *Uniform Terminology* as the language to translate each activity into a strategy for intervention has proven to be a positive tool for understanding the dimensions of activity. Throughout its three revisions, *Uniform Terminology* provided a structure for communicating in words how activity is used in intervention. Now rescinded, *Uniform Terminology* has been replaced by the *Occupational Therapy Practice Framework*. *Occupational Therapy Practice Framework* will continue to provide for and expand the language of our profession. The authors have collaborated to create a template for students with which they might grasp the basic concepts of activity analysis. This has been an evolutionary process taking place over the past 20 years and has led across confronting detours, diverse paths of thinking, and many avenues of debate. The end of the road has not been reached. This textbook is only an introduction in the clinical reasoning process. With experience and practice, this kind of analysis will become an automatic thinking pattern. "Activity analysis and syntheses... are then used to design therapeutic occupations to remediate the person's impairments that are limiting occupational performance" (Fisher, 1998, p. 519). Skills and abilities in clinical reasoning will grow through increasing contact with clients in delivering occupational therapy intervention. No one textbook, class, or professional degree fulfills the need for life-long learning. Education in this area will come through formal and informal learning situations, from continuing education workshops and conferences, from colleagues, professional literature, and, most of all, from clients.

Activity analysis and its application will remain one of the practitioner's most valuable assets in the future. As a profession, our potential has only begun to be realized. Returning to the basic beliefs in the power of occupation and purposeful activity has given added momentum to reach out to the community and reveal possibilities not dreamed of before. The writings of the recipients of the Eleanor Clarke Slagle Lectureship provide direction for the future of the profession. A striking aspect of these articles is the discrepancy between the findings of research and the limited scope of today's practice. Untapped population-based groups have needs that occupation-based intervention can fulfill. Areas such as the rise in the aging population, the focus on ergonomics, the assistive technology revolution, prevention practice arenas, the focus on addressing spirituality issues, and the constant change in medical treatment approaches are part of this potential. There are segments of the population of every community that are failing to realize the potential standards of health possible. The continued rate of abuse of drugs, chemicals, children, and spouses; the high rate of divorce, suicide, and violent crime; the presence of malnutrition, poverty, pollution, and unsatisfactory employment, all point to a pathology from which no community is immune (Gross & Moyer, 1977, p. 2). The health of the community is undeniably bound up with the health of the individuals residing in it (Rosenfeld, 1982, p. 235). A responsibility to address such areas is crucial, and practitioners must broaden their horizons to develop the many facets of that professional base called occupation. The challenge as a profession is to open the door to a wider view of how purposeful activity makes life worth living.

One way to meet this challenge is teaching the occupational therapy student the art and skill of making activity meaningful and purposeful. Further study in theory, frames of reference, treatment modalities, medical problems, and disabling conditions must be supplemented with problems facing the well population, health prevention, quality of life, and alleviation of barriers limiting the ability to function independently. Working from a knowledge founded on the intimate relationship between actively doing and health, the occupational therapy practitioner believes in the intrinsic value of goal-directed activity to attain a purpose in life and a sense of well-being (Sorensen, 1978, p. 288). Exploring and reflecting on the research and philosophy of such terms as *occupation, purposeful activity, function, independence,* and *health* results in a solid background and confidence to move forward into new practice arenas. The leadership of those from the past combined with the personal strengths and capabilities of today's practitioners will bring the profession into a strong tomorrow. As shown in the opening story, a difference in perspective can be the key.

REFERENCES

American Occupational Therapy Association. (1993). Position paper: Purposeful activity. *American Journal of Occupational Therapy, 47,* 1081-1082.

Fisher, A. G. (1998). Uniting practice and theory in an occupational framework: 1998 Eleanor Clarke Slagle Lecture. *American Journal of Occupational Therapy, 52*(7), 509-521.

Gross, D. M., & Moyer, E. A. (1977). *Occupational therapy in the community.* New York: New York State OT Association, Inc.

Rosenfeld, M. S. (1982). A model for activity intervention in disaster-stricken communities. *American Journal of Occupational Therapy, 36*(4), 229-235.

Sorensen, J. (1978). Occupational therapy in business: A new horizon. *American Journal of Occupational Therapy, 32*(5), 287-288.

West, W. (1973). The growing importance of prevention. In L. A. Llorens (Ed.), *Consultation in the community: Occupational therapy in child health.* Dubuque, Iowa: Kendall/Hunt.

Suggested Readings
Prior to 1996

Adelstein, L. A., & Nelson, D. L. (1985). Effects of sharing versus nonsharing on affective meaning in collage activities. *Occupational Therapy in Mental Health, 5, 29-45.*

Allen, C. (1982). Independence through activity: The practice of occupational therapy (psychiatry). *American Journal of Occupational Therapy, 36, 731-739.*

Allen, C. K. (1985). *OT for psychiatric diseases: Measurement and management of cognitive disabilities.* Boston, MA: Little, Brown & Co.

Allen, C. K., Earnart, C. A., & Blue, T. (1992). *Occupational therapy treatment goals for the physically and cognitively disabled.* Rockville, MD: AOTA.

Bakshi, R., Bhambhani, Y., & Madill, H. (1991). The effects of task preference on performance during purposeful and non-purposeful activities. *American Journal of Occupational Therapy, 45, 912-916.*

Banning, M. R., & Nelson, D. L. (1987). The effects of activity-elicited humor and group structure on group cohesion and affective meanings. *American Journal of Occupational Therapy, 41, 510-514.*

Bissell, J., & Mailloux, Z. (1981). The use of crafts in occupational therapy for the physically disabled. *American Journal of Occupational Therapy, 35, 369-374.*

Bloch, M., Smith, D., & Nelson, D. (1989). Heart rate, activity, duration, and affect in added-purpose versus single-purpose jumping activities. *American Journal of Occupational Therapy, 43, 25-29.*

Borst, & Nelson, D. L. (1993). Use of uniform terminology by occupational therapy students. *American Journal of Occupational Therapy, 47, 611.*

Breines, E. (2000). In times of bereavement. *Advance for Occupational Therapy Practitioners, March 13, 25.*

Breines, E. B. (1995). *Occupational therapy activities from clay to computers, theory and practice.* Philadelphia, PA: F. A. Davis Co.

Bundy, A. C. (1993). Assessment of play and leisure: Delineation of the problem. *American Journal of Occupational Therapy, 47* (3), 217-222.

Carter, B. A., Nelson, D. L., & Duncombe, L. W. (1983). The effect of psychological type on the mood and meaning of two collage activities. *American Journal of Occupational Therapy, 39, 688-693.*

Chandani, A., & Hill, C. (1990). What really is therapeutic activity? *British Journal of Occupational Therapy, 53, 15-18.*

Christiansen, C., & Baum, C. (1991). *Occupational therapy: Overcoming human performance deficits.* Thorofare, NJ: SLACK Incorporated.

Clark, P. N. (1979). Human development through occupation: Theoretical frameworks in contemporary occupational therapy practice. *American Journal of Occupational Therapy, 33, 505-514.*

Cottrell, R. P. F. (1996). *Perspectives on purposeful activity: Foundation and future of occupational therapy.* Bethesda, MD: AOTA.

DiJoseph, L. (1982). Independence through activity: Mind, body, and environment interaction in therapy. *American Journal of Occupational Therapy, 36, 740-744.*

Drake, M. (1999). *Crafts in therapy and rehabilitation, 2nd Ed.* Thorofare, NJ: SLACK Incorporated.

Dunn, W. (1982). Independence through activity: The practice of occupational therapy (pediatrics). *American Journal of Occupational Therapy, 36,* 745-747.

Dunn, W., Brown, C., & McGuigan, A. (1994). The ecology of human performance: A framework for considering the effect of context. *American Journal of Occupational Therapy, 48(7),* 595-607.

Dunn, W., & McGourty, L. (1989). Application of uniform terminology to practice. *American Journal of Occupational Therapy, 43,* 817-831.

Dunton, W. R. Jr. (1923). A debate upon toy-making as a therapeutic occupation: Con. *Archives of Occupational Therapy, 2,* 39-43.

Dunton, W. R. Jr. (1923). Rejoiner. *Archives of Occupational Therapy, 2,* 47.

Fahl, M. A. (1970). Emotionally disturbed children: Effects of cooperative and competitive activity on peer interaction. *American Journal of Occupational Therapy, 24,* 31-33.

Fidler, G. S. (1948). Psychological evaluation of occupational therapy activities. *American Journal of Occupational Therapy, 2,* 284-287.

Fidler, G. S. (1969). The task-oriented group as a context for treatment. *American Journal of Occupational Therapy, 23,* 43-48.

Fidler, G. S. (1981). From crafts to competence. *American Journal of Occupational Therapy, 35,* 567-573.

Fidler, G. S. (1996). Life-style performance: From profile to conceptual model. *American Journal of Occupational Therapy, 50* (2), 139-147.

Fidler, G. S., & Fidler, J. W. (1978). Doing and becoming: Purposeful action and self-actualization. *American Journal of Occupational Therapy, 32,* 305-310.

Fitts, H. A., & Howe, M. C. (1987). Use of leisure time by cardiac patients. *American Journal of Occupational Therapy, 41,* 583-589.

Fox, J., & Jirgal, D. (1967). Therapeutic properties of activities as examined by the clinical council of the Wisconsin schools of O.T. *American Journal of Occupational Therapy, 21,* 29-33.

Froehlich, J., & Nelson, D. L. (1986). Affective meanings of life review through activities and discussion. *American Journal of Occupational Therapy, 40,* 27-33.

Gliner, J. A. (1985). Purposeful activity in motor learning theory: An event approach to motor skill acquisition. *American Journal of Occupational Therapy, 39,* 28-34.

Grady, A. P. (1992). Occupation as vision. *American Journal of Occupational Therapy, 46* (12), 1062-1065.

Haase, B. (1995). Clinical interpretation of "occupationally embedded exercise versus rote exercise: A choice between occupational forms by elderly nursing home residents." *American Journal of Occupational Therapy, 49,* 403-404.

Hatter, J. K., & Nelson, D. L. (1987). Altruism and task participation in the elderly. *American Journal of Occupational Therapy, 41,* 379-381.

Henry, A. D., Nelson, D. L., & Duncombe, L. W. (1984). Choice-making in group and individual activity. *American Journal of Occupational Therapy, 38,* 245-251.

Hoover, J. A. B. (1996). Diversional occupational therapy in World War I: A need for purpose in occupations. *American Journal of Occupational Therapy, 50(10),* 881-885.

Huss, J. (1981). From kinesiology to adaptation. *American Journal of Occupational Therapy, 35,* 574-580.

Jacobshagen, I. (1990). The effect of interruption of activity of affect. *Occupational Therapy in Mental Health, 10(2),* 35-46.

Jongbloed, L., & Morgan, D. (1991). An investigation of involvement in leisure activities after a stroke. *American Journal of Occupational Therapy, 45,* 420-427.

Katz, N., & Cohen, E. (1991). Meanings ascribed to four craft activities before and after extensive learning. *Occupational Therapy Journal of Research, 11(1),* 24-39.

Kielhofner, G. (1980). A model of human occupation, Part 2. Ontogenesis perspective of temporal adaptation. *American Journal of Occupational Therapy, 34,* 657-663.

Kielhofner, G. (1980). A model of human occupation, Part 3. Benign and vicious cycles. *American Journal of Occupational Therapy, 34,* 731-737.

Kielhofner, G. (1982). A heritage of activity: Development of theory. *American Journal of Occupational Therapy, 36,* 723-730.

Kielhofner, G., & Burke, J. P. (1980). A model of human occupation, Part 1. Conceptual framework and content. *American Journal of Occupational Therapy, 34,* 572-581.

Kielhofner, G., Burke, J. P., & Igi, C. H. (1980). A model of human occupation, Part 4. Assessment and intervention. *American Journal of Occupational Therapy, 34,* 777-788.

Kircher, M. A. (1984). Motivation as a factor of perceived exertion in purposeful versus nonpurposeful activity. *American Journal of Occupational Therapy, 38,* 165-170.

Kleinman, B. L., & Stalcup, A. (1991). The effect of a graded craft activities on visuomotor integration in an inpatient child psychiatry population. *American Journal of Occupational Therapy, 45,* 324-330.

Kremer, E. R. H., Nelson, D. L., & Duncombe, L. W. (1984). Effects of selected activities on affective meaning in psychiatric clients. *American Journal of Occupational Therapy, 38,* 522-528.

Lang, E., Nelson, D., & Bush, M. (1992). Comparison of performance in materials-based occupation, imagery-based occupation, and rote exercise in nursing home residents. *American Journal of Occupational Therapy, 46,* 607-611.

Lerner, C. J. (1979). The magazine picture collage. *American Journal of Occupational Therapy, 33(8),* 500-504.

Levine, R. E., & Brayley, C. R. (1991). Occupation as a therapeutic medium: A contextual approach to performance intervention. In C. Christiansen, & C. Baum (Eds.), *Occupational therapy: Overcoming human performance deficits* (pp. 590-631). Thorofare, NJ: SLACK Incorporated.

Llorens, L. A. (1986). Activity analysis: Agreement among factors in a sensory processing model. *American Journal of Occupational Therapy, 40,* 103-110.

Lyon, B. G. (1983). Purposeful versus human activity. *American Journal of Occupational Therapy, 37,* 493-495.

Miller, L., & Nelson, D. L. (1987). Dual-purpose activity versus single-purpose activity in terms of duration on task, exertion level, and affect. *Occupational Therapy in Mental Health, 7,* 55-67.

Mullins, C. S., Nelson, D. L., & Smith, D. A. (1987). Exercise through dual-purpose activity in the institutionalized elderly. *Physical and Occupational Therapy in Geriatrics, 5,* 29-39.

Mumford, M. (1974). A comparison of interpersonal skills in verbal and activity groups. *American Journal of Occupational Therapy, 28,* 281-283.

Nelson, D. L. (1988). Occupation: Form and performance. *American Journal of Occupational Therapy, 42,* 633-641.

Nelson, D. L. (1996). Therapeutic occupation: A definition. *American Journal of Occupational Therapy, 50*(10), 775-782.

Nelson, D. L., & Peterson C. (1989). Enhancing therapeutic exercise through purposeful activity: A theoretic analysis. *Topics in Geriatric Rehabilitation, 4*(4), 12-22.

Nelson, D. L., Peterson C., Smith D. A., Boughton J. A., & Whalen G. M. (1988). Effects of project versus parallel groups on social interaction and affective responses in senior citizens. *American Journal of Occupational Therapy, 42,* 23-29.

Nelson, D. L., Thompson G., & Moore J. A. (1982). Identification of factors of affective meaning in four selected activities. *American Journal of Occupational Therapy, 36,* 381-387.

Niswander, P., & Hyde R. (1954). The value of crafts in psychiatric occupational therapy. *American Journal of Occupational Therapy, 8,* 104-106.

Peloquin, S. M. (1991). Occupational therapy service: Individual and collective understandings of the founders, Part 2. *American Journal of Occupational Therapy, 45,* 733-744.

Petrone, P. (1994). Clinical interpretation of "the relationship between occupational form and occupational performance: A kinematic perspective." *American Journal of Occupational Therapy, 48,* 688.

Pianetti, C., Palacios, M., & Elliott, L. (1964). Significance of color. *American Journal of Occupational Therapy, 18,* 137-140.

Polatajko, H. (1994). Dreams, dilemmas, and decisions for occupational therapy in the new millennium: A Canadian perspective. *American Journal of Occupational Therapy, 48,* 590-594.

Quiroga, V. A. M. (1995). *Occupational therapy: The first 30 years, 1900 to 1930.* Rockville, MD: AOTA.

Rocker, J. D., & Nelson, D. L. (1987). Affective responses to keeping and not keeping an activity product. *American Journal of Occupational Therapy, 41,* 152-157.

Rothaus, P., Hanson, P., & Cleveland, S. (1966). Art and group dynamics. *American Journal of Occupational Therapy, 20,* 182-187.

Royeen, C. B., Cynkin, S., & Robinson, A. M. (1990). Analyzing performance through activity. *AOTA Self Study Series: Assessing Function, No. 5.* Rockville, MD: AOTA.

Scardina, V. (1981). From pegboards to integration. *American Journal of Occupational Therapy, 35,* 581-588.

Schemm, R. (1994). Looking back: Bridging conflicting ideologies. The origins of American and British occupational therapy. *American Journal of Occupational Therapy, 48,* 1082-1087.

Shing-Ru Shih, L., Nelson, D. L., & Duncombe, L. W. (1984). Mood and affect following success and failure in two cultural groups. *Occupational Therapy Journal of Research, 4,* 213-230.

Shontz, F. C. (1959). Evaluation of psychological effects. *American Journal of Physical Medicine, 38,* 138-142.

Simon, C. J. (1993). Use of activity and activity analysis. In H. L. Hopkins, & H. D. Smith (Eds.), *Willard & Spackman's occupational therapy, 8th Ed.* (pp. 281-292). Philadelphia, PA: J. B. Lippincott Co.

Slade, S., Falkowski, W., Muwonge, A. K., & Slade, P. (1975). Immediate psychological effects of various occupational therapy activities on psychiatric patients: A pilot study. *British Journal of Occupational Therapy, 38,* 172-173.

Smith, P. A., Barrows, H. S., & Whitney, J. N. (1959). Psychological attributes of occupational therapy crafts. *American Journal of Occupational Therapy, 13,* 16-21, 25-26.

Steffan, J. A., & Nelson, D. L. (1987). The effects of tool scarcity on group climate and affective meaning within the context of a stenciling activity. *American Journal of Occupational Therapy, 41,* 449-453.

Steinbeck, T. M. (1986). Purposeful activity and performance. *American Journal of Occupational Therapy, 40,* 529-534.

Taber, F., Baron, S., & Blackwell, A. (1953). A study of a task directed and a free choice group. *American Journal of Occupational Therapy, 7,* 118-124.

Taylor, E., & Manguno, J. (1990). Use of treatment activities in occupational therapy. *American Journal of Occupational Therapy, 45*(4), 317-322.

Thibodeaux, D., & Ludwig, F. (1988). Intrinsic motivation in product-oriented and non-product-oriented activities. *American Journal of Occupational Therapy, 42,* 169-175.

Watson, D. E. (1997). *Task analysis: An occupational performance approach.* Bethesda, MD: AOTA.

Weston, D. L. (1960). Therapeutic crafts. *American Journal of Occupational Therapy, 14,* 121-123.

Weston, D. L. (1961). The dimensions of crafts. *American Journal of Occupational Therapy, 15,* 1-5.

Williamson, G. G. (1982). The heritage of activity: Development of theory. *American Journal of Occupational Therapy, 36,* 716-722.

Wood, W. (1995). Weaving the warp and weft of occupational therapy: An art and science for all times. *American Journal of Occupational Therapy, 49,* 44-52.

Wu, C., Trombly, C., & Lin, K. (1994). The relationship between occupational form and occupational performance: A kinematic perspective. *American Journal of Occupational Therapy, 48,* 679-687.

Yerxa, E. (1994). Dreams, dilemmas, and decisions for occupational therapy in the new millennium: An American perspective. *American Journal of Occupational Therapy, 48,* 586-589.

Yoder, R. M., Nelson, D. L., & Smith, D. A. (1989). Added-purpose versus rote exercise in female nursing home residents. *American Journal of Occupational Therapy, 43,* 581-586.

Zimmerer-Branum, S., & Nelson, D. (1995). Occupationally embedded exercise versus rote exercise: A choice between occupational forms by elderly nursing home residents. *American Journal of Occupational Therapy, 49,* 397-404.

Suggested Readings
From 1996 to 2003

AOTA Commission on Practice. (1998). Position paper: The use of general information and assistive technology within occupational therapy. *American Journal of Occupational Therapy, 52* (10), 870-71.

Baum, C. & Law, M. (1997). Occupational therapy practice: Focusing on occupational performance. *American Journal of Occupational Therapy, 51,* 277-288.

Bazyk, S., Stalnaker, D., Llerena, M., Ekelman, B., & Bazyk, J. (2003). Play in Mayan children. *American Journal of Occupational Therapy, 57*(3), 273-283.

Bober, S. J., Humphrey, R., Carswell, H. W., & Core, A. J. (2001). Toddlers' persistence in the emerging occupations of functional play and self-feeding. *American Journal of Occupational Therapy, 55*(4), 369-376.

Borell, L., Lilja, M., Sviden, G. A., & Sadlo, G. (2001). Occupations and signs of reduced hope: An explorative study of older adults with functional impairments. *American Journal of Occupational Therapy, 55*(3), 311-316.

Connor, M. (2000). Recreational folk dance: A multicultural exercise component in healthy ageing. *Australian Occupational Therapy Journal, 47*(2), 69-76.

Crabtree, J. (1998). The end of occupational therapy. *American Journal of Occupational Therapy, 52,* 205-214.

Crepeau, E. B. (1998). Activity analysis: A way of thinking about occupational performance. In M. E. Neistadt & E. B. Crepeau (Eds.), *Willard & Spackman's occupational therapy, 9th Ed.* pp. (135-147).

Crist, P. H., Davis, C. G., & Coffin, P. S. (2000). The employment and mental health status on the balance of work, play/leisure, self-care, and rest. *Occupational Therapy in Mental Health, 15*(1), 27-42.

Drake, M. (1992). *Crafts in therapy and rehabilitation.* Thorofare, NJ: SLACK Incorporated.

Ferguson, J. M., & Trombly, C. A. (1997). Effects of added purpose and meaningful occupation on motor learning. *American Journal of Occupational Therapy, 51*(7), 508-515.

Fisher, A. G. (1998). Uniting practice and theory in an occupational framework—1998 Eleanor Clarke Slagle Lecture. *American Journal of Occupational Therapy, 52*(7), 509-521.

Fisher, S. (2003). *The Canadian Occupational Performance Measure: Does it address the cultural occupations of ethnic minorities?* Medford, MA: Tufts University

Graham, S. F., & Bunrayong, W. (2002). Dance: A transformative occupation. *Journal of Occupational Science, 9*(3), 128-134.

Gray, J. M. (1998). Putting occupation into practice: Occupation as ends, occupation as means. *American Journal of Occupational Therapy, 52*(5), 354-364.

Hodgson, S., Lloyd, C., & Schmid, T. (2001). The leisure participation of clients with a dual diagnosis. *British Journal of Occupational Therapy, 64*(10), 487-492.

Howard, B. S. & J. R. (1997). Occupation as spiritual activity. *American Journal of Occupational Therapy, 51* (3), 181-185.

Howell, D., & Pierce, D. (2000). Exploring the forgotten restorative dimension of occupation: Quilting and quilt use. *Journal of Occupational Science, 7*(2), 68-72.

Iwarsson, S., Isacsson, A., Persson, D., & Schersten, B. (1998). Occupation and survival: A 25-year follow-up study of an aging population. *American Journal of Occupational Therapy, 52*(1), 65-70.

Jonsson, A. L. T., Moller, A., & Grimby, G. (1999). Managing occupations in everyday life to achieve adaptation. *American Journal of Occupational Therapy, 53*(4), 353-362.

Larson, E. A. (2000). The orchestration of occupation: The dance of mothers. *American Journal of Occupational Therapy, 54*(3), 269-280.

Law, M. (2002). Distinguished Scholar Lecture: Participation in the occupations of everyday life. *American Journal of Occupational Therapy, 56*(6), 640-649.

Lo, J. L., & Huang, S. L. (2000). Affective experiences during daily occupations: Measurement and results. *Occupational Therapy International, 7*(2), 134-144.

Magnus, E. (2001). Everyday occupations and the process of redefinition: A study of how meaning in occupation influences redefinition of identity in women with a disability. *Scandinavian Journal of Occupational Therapy, 8*(3), 115-124.

Nagel, M. J., & Rice, M. S. (2001). Cross-transfer effects in the upper extremity during an occupationally embedded exercise. *American Journal of Occupational Therapy, 55*(3), 317-323.

Nelson, D. L. (1997). Why the profession of occupational therapy will flourish in the 21st century: The 1996 Eleanor Clarke Slagle Lecture. *American Journal of Occupational Therapy, 51*(1), 11-24.

Paul, S., & Ramsey, D. (1998). The effects of electronic music-making as a therapeutic activity for improving upper extremity active range of motion. *Occupational Therapy International, 5*(3), 223-237.

Persson, D. (1996). Play and flow in an activity group: A case study of creative occupations with chronic pain patients. *Scandinavian Journal of Occupational Therapy, 3*(1), 33-42.

Pierce, D. (2001). Untangling occupation in activity. *American Journal of Occupational Therapy, 55*(2), 138-146.

Polatajko, H. (2001). The evolution of our occupational perspective: The journey from diversion through therapeutic use to enablement. *Canadian Journal of Occupational Therapy, 68*(4), 203-207.

Pratt, W. L., & Goodman, D. G. (1999). *Leisure occupations of community living adults 65+.* Bay Shore, NY: Touro College.

Primeau, L. A. (1998). Orchestration of work and play within families. *American Journal of Occupational Therapy, 52*(3), 188-195.

Rebeiro, K. L. (2001). Enabling occupation: The importance of an affirming environment. *Canadian Journal of Occupational Therapy, 68*(2), 80-89.

Segal, R. (2000). Adaptive Strategies of mothers with children with attention deficit hyperactivity disorder: Enfolding and unfolding occupations. *American Journal of Occupational Therapy, 54*(3), 300-306.

Spitzer, S. L. (2001). *No words necessary: An ethnography of daily activities with young children who don't talk.* Los Angeles: University of Southern California.

Thomas, J. J. (1996). Materials-based, imagery-based, and rote exercise occupational forms: Effect on repetitions, heart rate, duration of performance, and self-perceived rest period on well elderly women. *American Journal of Occupational Therapy, 50*(10), 783-789.

Vrkljan, B., & Miller-Polgar, J. (2001). Meaning of occupational engagement in life-threatening illness: A qualitative pilot project. *Canadian Journal of Occupational Therapy, 68*(4), 237-246.

Wikstrom, I., Isacsson, A., & Jacobsson, L. T. H. (2001). Leisure activities in rheumatoid arthritis: Change after disease onset and associated factors. *British Journal of Occupational Therapy, 64*(2), 87-92.

Yerxa, E. J. (1998). Health and the human spirit for occupation. *American Journal of Occupational Therapy, 52*(6), 412-418.

Appendices

Appendix A

Position Papers of the American Occupational Therapy Association

Please note that Position Paper: Occupational Performance *and* Position Paper: Purposeful Activity *are presented for historical significance only. They have been rescinded by the American Occupational Therapy Association.*

POSITION PAPER: OCCUPATION

Concern with the occupational nature of human beings was fundamental to the establishment of occupational therapy. Since the time of occupational therapy's founding, the term occupation has been used to refer to an individual's active participation in self-maintenance, work, leisure, and play (American Occupational Therapy Association [AOTA], 1993; Bing, 1981; Levine, 1991; Meyer, 1922). Within the literature of the field, however, the meaning of occupation has been ambiguous because the term has been used interchangeably with other concepts. This paper's intent is to distinguish the term occupation from other terms, to summarize traditional beliefs about its nature and therapeutic value, and to identify factors that have impeded the study and discussion of occupation.

The Dynamic, Multidimensional Nature of Occupations

Occupations are the normal and familiar things that people do every day. This simple description reflects, but understates, the multidimensional and complex nature of daily occupation.

Occupations can be broadly explained as having both performance and contextual dimensions because they involve acts within defined settings (Christiansen, 1991; Nelson, 1988; Rogers, 1982). In that they frequently extend over time, occupations have a temporal dimension (Kielhofner, 1977; Meyer, 1922). Further, in that engagement in occupation is seen to be driven by an intrinsic need for mastery, competence, self-identity, and group acceptance, occupations have a psychological dimension (Brown, 1986; Burke, 1977; Christiansen, 1994; DiMatteo, 1991; Fidler & Fidler, 1979, 1983; White, 1971). Since occupations are often associated with a social or occupational role and are therefore identifiable in the culture, they have social and symbolic dimensions (Fidler & Fidler, 1983; Frank, 1994; Mosey, 1986). Finally, because they are infused with meaning within the lives of individuals, occupations have spiritual dimensions (Clark, 1993; Mattingly & Fleming, 1993). The term spiritual is used here to refer to the nonphysical and nonmaterial aspects of existence. In this sense, it is postulated that daily pursuits contribute insight into the nature and meaning of a person's life.

This multidimensional view of occupations and their central place in the experience of living was recognized early in the profession's history. Influenced by the pragmatic philosophies of John Dewey and William James (Breines, 1987), which related well-being to an individual's participation in the world around him or her, early theorists such as Tracy (1910), Dunton (1918), and Slagle (1922) contended that doing things favorably influenced interest and attention, provided relaxation, promoted moral development, reenergized the individual, normalized habits, and conferred a physical benefit (Upham, 1918).

Adolph Meyer (1922) asserted that, for healthy people, daily living unfolds in a natural and balanced pattern of occupational pursuits that bring both satisfaction and fulfillment. He noted that occupations have a performance or doing component, as well as a spiritual or personal meaning component. Meyer recognized that through daily occupations, people organized their lives in terms of time and made meaning of their existence as human beings. Meyer believed that the organizing, self-fulfilling characteristics of occupations could make them an important mechanism of adaptation. He postulated that the individual could affect his or her state of health through occupations selected and performed each day. This view has been a principle of many conceptual frames of reference developed by occupational therapy scholars since that time (Christiansen, 1991; Kielhofner, 1993; Reilly, 1962).

In summary, occupational therapy scholars agree that human occupations have emotional, cognitive, physical, spiritual, and contextual dimensions, all of which are related to general well-being. However, occupational therapy scholars have not been able to agree on the specific concepts regarding these dimensions, or on specific terms to name them.

Distinguishing Between Occupation and Related Terms

The physical and mental abilities and skills required for satisfactory engagement in a given occupational pursuit constitute the performance dimension of human occupation, often referred to in the occupational therapy literature as occupational performance. The performance dimension of occupations is that aspect which has received the most study and attention in the history of the field. This may explain why the terms function and purposeful activity have been used as synonyms for engagement in occupation (Henderson et al., 1991).

Occupations, because of their intentional nature, always involve mental abilities and skills, and typically, but not always, have an observable physical or active dimension. Whether one is laying bricks or practicing meditation exercises, one can be said to be "doing" something. Only one of these occupations, however, requires observable physical action. Whether physical or mental in nature, the behaviors necessary for completion of tasks in daily occupations can be analyzed according to specific components related to moving, perceiving, thinking, and feeling. Various occupational performance components have been described and defined within the *Uniform Terminology for Occupational Therapy, Third Edition* (AOTA, 1994).

Position papers on function and purposeful activity have been developed by the AOTA, and it is important to clarify the differences in meaning between these terms and the term occupation. The AOTA has proposed that when occupational therapists use the term function, they refer to an individual's performance of activities, tasks, and roles during daily occupations (occupational performance) (AOTA, 1995). Purposeful activity has also been recognized as a term to describe engagement in the tasks of daily living, with the use of this term emphasizing the intentional, goal directed nature of such engagement (AOTA, 1993). In this paper, it is proposed that reference to human occupation necessarily encompasses the required human capacities to act on the environment with intentionality in a given pursuit, as well as the unique organization of these pursuits over time and the meanings attributed to them by doers as well as those observing them.

In summary, occupations have performance, contextual, temporal, psychological, social, symbolic, and spiritual dimensions; whereas function in its specific use denotes primarily the performance dimension. While the term purposeful activity recognizes multiple dimensions and emphasizes intentionality, it is viewed as a term that does not capture the richness of human enterprise embodied in the word occupation. It is asserted that while all occupations constitute purposeful activity, not all purposeful activities can be described as occupations.

Therapeutic Benefits of Occupations

Since Adolph Meyer's (1922) philosophical essay, many scholarly papers have been written about the therapeutic value of occupations (Clark, 1993; Cynkin & Robinson, 1990; Englehardt, 1977; Reilly, 1962; Yerxa, 1967). These have identified a broad scope of benefits, ranging from the facilitation of habilitation, adaptation, and self-actualization to improvements in motor control and sensory processing. While there is growing evidence to support some of these claims, additional research is needed before it can be demonstrated that other benefits are likely valid.

Because occupation is an extremely complex phenomenon and has not been subjected to rigorous research until recently, many questions about its nature and its relationship to health and well-being remain unanswered. This emphasizes the need for further study. Current beliefs and theories about occupation should be regarded as incomplete and evolving.

Forces Advancing and Impeding the Study and Discussion of Occupation

One of the problems inhibiting the study of occupations is how to clearly, logically, and consistently describe different levels and types of occupations. Used here, the term levels refers to the complexity of a given occupation. For example, while getting dressed and driving to work are readily interpretable as organized sets of actions that may partially comprise a typical day, each of these involves a variety of specific and definable behaviors, such as buttoning a shirt or turning an ignition key, which are less complex. Even occupational behaviors of greater complexity, such as dressing or driving, are nested within clusters of activity that comprise and are recognized as part of larger sets of organized behavior within cultures, such as pursuing a career. This phenomenon of nesting, where simple acts can be identified as parts of more complex sets of acts, is a dimension of occupations that relates to their organization over time and can be viewed as reflecting varying levels of complexity.

The English language has words associated with occupations, such as actions, tasks, and projects, which imply differences in complexity. Evans (1987) and Kielhofner (1993) have been among those who have described the hierarchical nature of occupations, and others (Christiansen, 1991; Nelson, 1988) have suggested that it would be useful if specific terms for human enterprise denoted different levels of this

hierarchy. However, there is little agreement among scholars in occupational therapy or in the social sciences for how these terms ought to be used to describe varying levels of complexity in occupational behavior.

Similar difficulties exist in describing types or categories of occupations. Certain categories of occupations have gained conventional usage by occupational therapists and are recognized in contemporary culture. These include work, self-care (or maintenance), play, and leisure.

Studies of human beings in different cultures have shown similarities in time use according to these general categories (Christiansen, in press). However, while general categories of occupations are recognized across cultures, the specific tasks that constitute each category and the delineation of categories vary across individuals. The classification of a given task within a larger category seems to be dependent upon the context in which it is performed. For example, sewing may be viewed as work by some and classified as leisure by others.

Similarly, most occupational pursuits seem to have both a general or cultural meaning attributed by participants and observers as well as a specific and personal meaning known only to the performer (Nelson, 1988; Rommerveit, 1980). Consider, for example, that getting dressed is viewed as a necessary and practical aspect of daily life in most cultures, but assumes symbolic importance when it is performed without assistance for the first time by the 3-year-old child, or by an adult mastering use of a new prosthetic arm. Dressing in anticipation of a ceremony or developmental milestone, such as high school graduation or a wedding, imbues the act with special significance. Over time, the experiences embedded in daily occupations assume collective meaning and are interpreted as essential part of a person's self-narrative or life story (Bruner, 1990; Clark, 1993; Mattingly & Fleming, 1993).

Research on Occupations and Research in Occupational Therapy

It is useful to recognize that research on occupations should be distinguished from research in occupational therapy (Mosey, 1992). In the first instance, inquiry is directed toward understanding the nature of the typical daily occupations in which people engage; that is, what people do, how they do it, and why they do it. The study of occupational therapy, conversely, concerns itself with the effect of occupation on health, development of frames of reference that facilitate the identification and remediation of occupational dysfunction, and other topical issues of significance to this science-based profession.

Research for both areas has been impeded by the lack of conventional definitions for terms related to occupation. This, in turn, has contributed to disagreements about the proper concern of practice and the appropriate focus of research (Christiansen, 1981, 1991; Kielhofner & Burke, 1977; Mosey, 1985, 1989; Rogers, 1982; Shannon, 1977). Recently, occupational science has emerged as an area of study concerned with understanding humans as occupational beings (Clark et al., 1991; Yerxa et al., 1989). As additional research enables us to learn more about the nature of occupations and their potential as a means for promoting and restoring health and well-being, it is likely that there will be continued discussion on the use of terminology to describe specific concepts.

This paper has attempted to identify distinctions among current terms related to human occupation. As our understanding of occupations advances, more concepts and terms will evolve. It is important to continue to develop knowledge about occupations to facilitate our further understanding of an important, complex, and rich aspect of human life. In this way, the profession of occupational therapy will better appreciate the vision of its founders, more clearly understand its current state, and more likely realize the potential embodied in occupations as touchstones of human existence.

REFERENCES

American Occupational Therapy Association. (1993). Position paper: Purposeful activity. *American Journal of Occupational Therapy, 47*, 1081-1082.

American Occupational Therapy Association. (1994). Uniform terminology for occupational therapy—Third edition. *American Journal of Occupational Therapy, 48*, 1047-1059.

American Occupational Therapy Association. (1995). Position paper: Occupational performance: Occupational therapy's definition of function. *American Journal of Occupational Therapy, 49*, 1019-1020.

Bing, R. (1981). Occupational therapy revisited: A paraphrastic journey. *American Journal of Occupational Therapy, 35*, 499-518.

Breines, E. (1987). Pragmatism as a foundation for occupational therapy. *American Journal of Occupational Therapy, 41*, 522-525.

Brown, R. (1986). *Social psychology* (2nd ed.). New York: Free Press.

Bruner, J. (1990). *Acts of Meaning.* Cambridge, MA: Harvard University Press.

Burke, J. P. (1977). A clinical perspective on motivation: Pawn versus origin. *American Journal of Occupational Therapy, 31*, 254-258.

Christiansen, C. (1981). Toward resolution of crisis: Research requisites in occupational therapy. *Occupational Therapy Journal of Research, 1*, 115-124.

Christiansen, C. (1991). Occupational therapy: Intervention for life performance. In C. Christiansen & C. Baum (Eds.), *Occupational therapy: Overcoming human performance deficits* (pp. 1-13). Thorofare, NJ: SLACK Incorporated.

Christiansen, C. (1994). A social framework for understanding self-care intervention. In C. Christiansen (Ed.), *Ways of living: Self-care strategies for special needs* (pp. 1-26). Rockville, MD: American Occupational Therapy Association.

Christiansen, C. (In press). Three perspectives on balance in occupation. In F. Clark & R. Zemke (Eds.), *Occupational science: The first five years.* Philadelphia: F. A. Davis.

Clark, F. A. (1993). Occupation embedded in a real life: Interweaving occupational science and occupational therapy. 1993 Eleanor Clarke Slagle Lecture. *American Journal of Occupational Therapy, 47*, 1067-1078.

Clark, F. A., Parham, D., Carlson, M. E., Frank, G., Jackson, J., Pierce, D., Wolfe, R. J., & Zemke, R. (1991). Occupational science: Academic innovation in the service of occupational therapy's future. *American Journal of Occupational Therapy, 45*, 300-310.

Cynkin, S., & Robinson, A. M. (1990). *Occupational therapy and activities health: Toward health through activities.* Boston: Little, Brown.

DiMatteo, M. R. (1991). *The psychology of health, illness, and medical care: An individual perspective.* Pacific Grove, CA: Brooks-Cole.

Dunton, W. R. (1918). The principles of occupational therapy. *Public Health Nurse, 10*, 316-321.

Englehardt, H. T. (1977). Defining occupational therapy: The meaning of therapy and the virtues of occupation. *American Journal of Occupational Therapy, 31*, 666-672.

Evans, A. K. (1987). Nationally speaking: Definition of occupation as the core concept of occupational therapy. *American Journal of Occupational Therapy, 41*, 627-628.

Fidler, G. S. (1981). From crafts to competence. *American Journal of Occupational Therapy, 35*, 567-573.

Fidler, G. S. & Fidler, J. W. (1979). Doing and becoming: Purposeful action and self-actualization. *American Journal of Occupational Therapy, 32*, 305-310.

Fidler, G. S., & Fidler, J. W. (1983). Doing and becoming: The occupational therapy experience. In G. Kielhofner (Ed.), *Health through occupation* (pp. 267-280). Philadelphia: F.A. Davis.

Frank, G. (1994). The personal meaning of self-care. In C. Christiansen (Ed.), *Ways of living: Self-care strategies for special needs* (pp. 27-49). Rockville, MD: American Occupational Therapy Association.

Henderson, A., Cermak, S., Coster, W., Murray, E., Trombly, C., & Tickle-Degnen, L. (1991). The issue is: Occupational science is multidimensional. *American Journal of Occupational Therapy, 45*, 370-372.

Kielhofner, G. (1977). Temporal adaptation: A conceptual framework for occupational therapy. *American Journal of Occupational Therapy, 31*, 235-242.

Kielhofner, G. (1993). *Conceptual foundations of occupational therapy.* Philadelphia: F. A. Davis.

Kielhofner, G., & Burke, J. P. (1977). Occupational therapy after sixty years: An account of changing identity and knowledge. *American Journal of Occupational Therapy, 31*, 675-689.

Levine, R. (1991). Occupation as a therapeutic medium. In C. Christiansen & C. Baum (Eds.), *Occupational therapy: Overcoming human performance deficits* (pp. 592-631). Thorofare, NJ: SLACK Incorporated.

Mattingly, C., & Fleming, M. (1993). *Clinical reasoning.* Philadelphia: F.A. Davis.

Meyer, A. (1922). The philosophy of occupational therapy. *Archives of Occupational Therapy, 1*, 1-10.

Mosey, A. C. (1985). A monistic or pluralistic approach to professional identity. *American Journal of Occupational Therapy, 39*, 504-509.

Mosey, A. C. (1986). *Psychosocial components of occupational therapy.* New York: Raven.

Mosey, A. C. (1989). The proper focus of scientific inquiry in occupational therapy: Frames of reference. *Occupational Therapy Journal of Research, 9*, 195-201.

Mosey, A. C. (1992). Partition of occupational science and occupational therapy. *American Journal of Occupational Therapy, 46*, 851-855.

Nelson, D. L. (1988). Occupation: Form and performance. *American Journal of Occupational Therapy, 42*, 633-641.

Reilly, M. (1962). Occupation can be one of the great ideas of 20th century medicine. *American Journal of Occupational Therapy, 16*, 1-9.

Rogers, J. (1982). The spirit of independence: The evolution of a philosophy. *American Journal of Occupational Therapy, 36*, 709-715.

Rommerveit, R. (1980). On meanings of acts and what is meant and made known by what is said in a pluralistic social world. In M. Brenner (Ed.), *The structure of action* (pp. 108-149). Oxford: Basil Blackwell.

Shannon, P. D. (1977). The derailment of occupational therapy. *American Journal of Occupational Therapy, 31*, 229-234.

Slagle, E. C. (1922). Training aids for mental patients. *Archives of Occupational Therapy, 1*, 11-17.

Tracy, S. (1910). *Studies in invalid occupations: A manual for nurses and attendants.* Boston: Whitcomb & Burrows.

Upham, E. G. (1918). *Ward occupations in hospitals.* Federal Board for Vocational Education Bulletin 25. Washington, DC: Government Printing Office.

White, R. W. (1971). The urge towards competence. *American Journal of Occupational Therapy, 25*, 271-274.

Yerxa, E. (1967). Authentic occupational therapy. *American Journal of Occupational Therapy, 21*, 1-9.

Yerxa, E., Clark, F., Frank, G., Jackson, J., Parham, D., Pierce, D., Stein, C., & Zemke, R. (1989). An introduction to occupational science: A foundation for occupational therapy in the 21st century. In J. Johnson & E. Yerxa (Eds.), *Occupational science: The foundation for new models of practice* (pp. 1-18). New York: Haworth.

Prepared by Charles Christiansen, EdD, OTR, OT(C), FAOTA; Florence Clark, PhD, OTR, FAOTA; Gary Kielhofner, DPM, OTR, FAOTA; Joan Rogers, PhD, OTR, FAOTA; with contributions from David Nelson, PhD, OTR, FAOTA for the Commission on Practice (Jim Hinojosa, PhD, OTR, FAOTA, Chairperson). Adopted by the Representative Assembly 1995.

POSITION PAPER: PURPOSEFUL ACTIVITY

The American Occupational Therapy Association (AOTA) submits this paper to clarify the use of the term purposeful activity, a central focus of occupational therapy throughout its history. People engage in purposeful activity as part of their daily life routines in the context of occupational performance (AOTA, 1979). Occupation refers to active participation in self-maintenance, work, leisure, and play. Purposeful activity refers to goal-directed behaviors or tasks that comprise occupations. An activity is purposeful if the individual is an active, voluntary participant and if the activity is directed toward a goal that the individual considers meaningful (Evans, 1987; Gilfoyle, 1984; Mosey, 1986; Nelson, 1988). The purposefulness of an activity lies with the individual performing the activity and with the context in which it is done (Henderson et al., 1991). The meaning of an activity is unique to each person, influenced by his or her life experiences (Mosey, 1986; Pedretti, 1982), life roles, interests, age, and cultural background, as well as the situational context in which the activity occurs. Occupational therapy practitioners (i.e., registered occupational therapists and certified occupational therapy assistants) are committed to the use of purposeful activity to evaluate, facilitate, restore, or maintain individuals' abilities to function in their daily occupations.

Occupational therapists use activities to evaluate an individual's capacities to meet the functional demands of his or her environment and daily life. On the basis of an evaluation, the occupational therapy practitioner, in collaboration with the individual, designs activity experiences that offer the individual opportunities for effective action. Purposeful activities assist and build upon the individual's abilities and lead to achievement of personal functional goals.

Purposeful activity provides opportunities for persons to achieve mastery of their environment, and successful performance promotes feelings of personal competence (Fidler & Fidler, 1978). A person who is involved in purposeful activity directs attention to the goal rather than to the processes required for achievement of the goal. Engagement in purposeful activity within the context of interpersonal, cultural, physical, and other environmental conditions requires and elicits coordination among the individual's sensory motor, cognitive, and psychosocial systems. Purposeful activity may involve the independent use of complex cognitive processes, such as premeditation, reflection, planning, and use of symbolic cues. Conversely, it may involve less complex processes and take place in an environment of external structure, support, and supervision (Allen, 1987; Henderson et al., 1991). Engagement in purposeful activity provides direct and objective feedback of performance both to the occupational therapy practitioner and the individual.

The therapeutic purposes for which purposeful activity is used include mastery of a new skill, restoration of a deficient ability, compensation for functional disability, health maintenance, or prevention of dysfunction. To use purposeful activity therapeutically, an occupational therapy practitioner analyzes the activity from several perspectives. First, the activity is examined to identify its component parts to determine which skills and abilities are necessary to complete the task. Second, it is examined in terms of the context in which it will be performed. Third, the practitioner considers the person's age, occupational roles, cultural background, gender, interests, and preferences that may influence the meaningfulness of the activity for the individual. All this information is considered together to assist the occupational therapy practitioner in synthesizing (i.e., adapting, grading, and combining) activities for therapeutic purposes for a particular individual.

Purposeful activities cannot be prescribed on the basis of analysis of their inherent characteristics alone; rather, by definition, prescription of purposeful activity is individual-specific. An occupational therapy practitioner grades or adapts a chosen activity for an individual to promote successful performance or elicit a particular response. Grading activities challenges the patient's abilities by progressively changing the process, tools, materials, or environment of a given activity to gradually increase or decrease performance demands. These incremental modifications are made in response to the individual's dynamic changes and provide opportunities for gradual development of skill and related therapeutic benefits. The grading of activities is accomplished by modifying the sequence, duration, or procedures of the task; the individual's position; the position of the tools and materials; the size, shape, weight, or texture of the materials; the nature and degree of interpersonal contact; the extent of physical handling by the occupational therapy practitioner during performance; or the environment in which the activity is attempted. Supportive or assistive devices or techniques may be used to enhance the effectiveness of an activity or to facilitate performance (Henderson et al., 1991; Pedretti & Pasquinelli, 1990). Such techniques or devices are considered facilitative or preparatory to performance of purposeful activity and engagements in occupations.

If the therapy goal is to enhance a performance component so that an individual can engage in an occupational performance area, the selected activity and environmental conditions are manipulated to present graded challenges to the specific skills required. When an individual's successful completion of a task is a priority, occupational therapy practitioners adapt the task and the environment to facilitate performance. Adaptation is a process that changes an aspect of the activity or the environment to enable successful performance and accomplish a particular therapeutic goal. Adaptation of a task may require the use of assistive devices and techniques or grading strategies.

Occupational therapy education provides the necessary background for using activities as therapeutic modalities by instructing the student about behavioral and biological sciences related to the use and meaning of activity, about the nature of purposeful activity, and about the application of activity to therapeutic problems within occupational therapy frames of reference.

In summary, purposeful activity occurs within the context of work, self-care, play, and leisure activities and is used therapeutically to evaluate, facilitate, restore, or maintain individuals' abilities to function competently within their daily occupations. The occupational therapy practitioner's commitment to those whom he or she serves is to guide them in the use of purposeful activities so as to empower them to enhance the quality of their being in the daily reality where they live as parents, children, students, homemakers, workers, or retirees (Reilly, 1966).

REFERENCES

Allen, C. K. (1987). Activity: Occupational therapy's treatment method (Slagle lecture). *American Journal of Occupational Therapy, 41*, 563-575.

American Occupational Therapy Association. (1979). Resolution C, 531-79: The philosophical base of occupational therapy. *American Journal of Occupational Therapy, 33*, 785.

Evans, K. A. (1987). Nationally speaking—Definition of occupation as the core concept of occupational therapy. *American Journal of Occupational Therapy, 41*, 627-628.

Fidler, G. S., & Fidler, J. W. (1978). Doing and becoming: Purposeful action and self-actualization. *American Journal of Occupational Therapy, 38*, 305-310.

Gilfoyle, E. M. (1984). Transformation of a profession (Slagle lecture). *American Journal of Occupational Therapy, 38*, 575-584.

Henderson, A., Cermak, S., Coster, W., Murray, E., Trombly, C., & Tickle-Degnen, L. (1991). The issue is—Occupational science is multidimensional. *American Journal of Occupational Therapy, 45*, 370-372.

Mosey, A. C. (1986). *Psychosocial components of occupational therapy.* New York, NY: Raven.

Nelson, D. L. (1988). Occupation: Form and performance. *American Journal of Occupational Therapy, 42*, 633-641.

Pedretti, L. W. (1982, May). The compatibility of current treatment methods in physical disabilities with the philosophical base of occupational therapy. Paper presented at the 62nd Annual Conference of the American Occupational Therapy Association, Philadelphia, PA.

Pedretti, L. W., & Pasquinelli, S. (1990). A frame of reference for occupational therapy in physical dysfunction. In L. W. Pedretti & B. Zoltan (Eds.), *Occupational therapy practical skills for physical dysfunction* (pp. 1-17). St. Louis, MO: Mosby.

Reilly, M. (1966). The challenge of the future to an occupational therapist. *American Journal of Occupational Therapy, 20,* 221-225.

Prepared by Jim Hinojosa, PhD, OTR, FAOTA; Joyce Sabari, PhD, OTR; and Lorraine Pedretti, MS, OTR, with contributions from Mark S. Rosenfeld, PhD, OTR and Catherine Trombly, ScD, OTR/L, FAOTA, for the Commission on Practice (Jim Hinojosa, PhD, OTR, FAOTA, Chairperson).

Approved by the Representative Assembly April 1983. Revised and approved by the Representative Assembly June 1993.

POSITION PAPER: OCCUPATIONAL PERFORMANCE: OCCUPATIONAL THERAPY'S DEFINITION OF FUNCTION

Fidler and Fidler (1963) define function as "doing"; Trombly (1993) promotes the use of "occupational function"; and function can describe a performance (i.e., functional strength, functional range of motion, and functional skills). The word function can mean role, use, activity, capacity, job, position, pursuit, or place (Landau & Bogus, 1977). The many ways in which the word function is used, or implied, may contribute to confusion regarding occupational therapy's unique role in addressing function. Although there may be some confusion about the use of terms, there is no confusion about the sense of purpose held by occupational therapy practitioners as they address the functional needs of the clients they serve.

Occupational therapy uses the word function interchangeably with performance and occupational performance because occupation therapy's domain is the function of the person in his or her occupational roles. The concept of function is implicit, rather than explicit, in many of the frames of reference used by occupational therapy practitioners as they focus on strategies to overcome deficits that impair the function of the individual. Occupational therapy practitioners help people address challenges or difficulties that threaten or impair their ability to perform activities and tasks that are basic to the fulfillment of their roles as worker, parent, spouse or partner, sibling, and friend to self or others.

In order to understand how occupational therapy uses function, it is necessary to review the historical roots of occupational therapy. Occupational therapy emerged az a developing profession in the years during and following World War I. The theoretical writings of Adolph Meyer (1922) and others were initially influenced by the then emerging school of American psychology whose "functional approach" focused on the process of adaptation to the environment rather than to the structure of the organism (Boring, 1950). The founders of occupational therapy were committed to the importance of occupation and the preservation of function (Peloquin, 1991), and early clinical efforts focused on the role of work and productivity to maintain or improve function (Hopkins, 1988). The concept of function and occupation remains at the core of occupational therapy today. However, more recently, the interaction of the functional and structural approaches has emerged, and function is viewed as the interaction of neural and physiological mechanisms, behavior, and environment. This interaction is critical to understanding the effect of occupation on health (Almli, 1993), as the function of the individual is supported in a dynamic relationship between the person, his or her occupation, and the environment (see Figure 1). The unique term used by occupational therapies to express function is occupational performance. "Occupational performance reflects the individual's dynamic experience of engaging in daily occupations within the environment" (Law & Baum, 1994, p. 12).

The concept of function has always been a central focus of occupational therapy and remains so. Other professions are beginning to recognize its importance and are placing increased value on function. Fisher (1992) acknowledged that the common goal of promoting functional independence is shared by occupational therapy, physical therapy, nursing, social work, psychology, and medicine, among others. A shift is occurring from a focus on pathology to a focus on function, as one of the primary indicators of treatment effectiveness (Ware, 1993). This shift also brings to the forefront the issues that occupational therapy has always valued—the person's capacity to function in a community context.

Occupational therapy's emphasis on function is broader than the function of a human organ [or body part] (Christiansen, 1991). It goes far beyond the loss or abnormality of the anatomical structure or function as defined by impairment (National Center for Medical Rehabilitation Research [NCMRR], 1993); or the lack of ability to perform and action or activity in the manner considered normal as defined by functional limitation (NCMRR, 1993). Occupational therapy views the individual as performing activities and roles within a social, cultural, and physical environment as defined by ability, or with a limitation—disability (NCMRR, 1993). The occupational therapy practitioner addresses the function of the individual at the occupational performance level where the environmental supports and barriers, the individual's skills, and the individual's occupational demands interact (see Figure 2).

Since 1917, occupational therapy has focused its services to enhance the function of individuals with, or threatened with, disability. Its practitioners have focused their efforts on function by using interventions to improve the occupational performance of persons who lack the ability to perform an action or activity considered necessary for their everyday lives. This is accomplished through a joint effort of the person and the clinician, where the person's problems, strengths, and assets are identified; followed by therapeutic interventions, educational strategies, access to resources, and environmental adaptations, so the person can accomplish his or her goals (Law & Baum, 1994). The unique contribution of occupational therapy is that the practitioner creates the opportunity for individuals to gain the skill and confidence to accomplish activities and tasks that are meaningful and productive, and in doing so, increases their occupational performance, thus their function.

REFERENCES

Almli, C. R. (1993, June). *Motor system, development, and neuroplasticity: Implications of theory and practice in occupational therapy.* AOTF Research Colloquium, Seattle, WA.

Boring, E. G. (1950). *A history of experimental psychology* (2nd ed.). Englewood Cliffs, NJ: Prentice Hall.

Christiansen, C. (1991). Occupational therapy intervention for life performance. In C. Christiansen & C. M. Baum (Eds.), *Occupational therapy: Overcoming human performance deficits* (pp. 3-43). Thorofare, NJ: SLACK Incorporated.

Fidler, G., & Fidler, J. (1963). *Occupational therapy: A communication process in psychiatry.* New York: Macmillan.

Fisher, A. G. (1992). The Foundation—Functional measures, part 1: What is function, what should we measure, and how should we measure it? *American Journal of Occupational Therapy, 46,* 183-185.

Hopkins, H. L. (1988). An historical perspective on occupational therapy. In H. L. Hopkins & H. D. Smith (Eds.), *Willard and Spackman's occupational therapy* (7th ed., pp. 16-37). Philadelphia, PA: Lippincott.

Landau, S. L., & Bogus, R. J. (1977). *The Doubleday Roget's thesaurus in dictionary form* (p. 278). Garden City, NY: Doubleday.

Law, M., & Baum, C. M. (1994). *Creating the future: A Joint effort.* St. Louis: Authors (Program in Occupational Therapy, Washington University School of Medicine, 4567 Scott Avenue, St. Louis, MO 63110).

Meyer, A. (1922). The philosophy of occupational therapy. *Archives of Occupational Therapy, 1*(1), 1-10.

National Center for Medical Rehabilitation. Research. (1993). Research Plan for the National Center for Medical Rehabilitation Research (National Institutes of Health Publication No. 93 - 3509). Washington, DC: U.S. Government Printing Office.

Peloquin, S. M. (1991). Looking Back—Occupational therapy service: Individual and collective understanding of the founders, part 1. *American Journal of Occupational Therapy, 45,* 352-360.

Trombly, C. (1993). The Issue Is—Anticipating the future: Assessment of occupational function. *American Journal of Occupational Therapy, 47,* 253-257.

Ware, J. E. (1993). Measures for a new era of health assessment. In A. L. Stewart & J. E. Ware (Eds.), *Measuring functioning and well-being* (pp. 3-12). Durham, NC: Duke University Press.

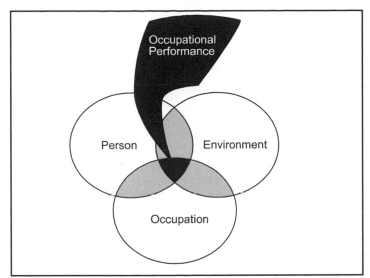

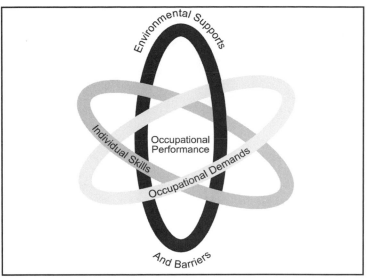

Figure 1. Reprinted with permission from Law, M. (1993). Planning for children with physical disabilities: Identifying and changing disabling environments through participatory research. Doctoral dissertation, University of Waterloo, Waterloo, Canada.

Figure 2. Reprinted with permission from Law, M., Cooper, B., Letts, L., Rigby, P., Stewart, S., & Strong, S. (1994). A model of person-environment interactions: Application to occupational therapy. Unpublished manuscript, McMaster University, Hamilton, Canada.

Prepared by Carolyn Baum, PhD, OTR, FAOTA; Dorothy Edwards, PhD; and the faculty of the Program in Occupational Therapy, Washington University School of Medicine, St. Louis, MO, for the Commission on Practice (Jim Hinojosa, PhD, OTR, FAOTA, Chairperson).

Adopted by the Representative Assembly April 1995.

Appendix B

Uniform Terminology for Reporting Occupational Therapy Services, First Edition

Please note that this document is presented for historical significance only. It has been rescinded by the American Occupational Therapy Association.

INTRODUCTION

August 1978, the American Occupational Therapy Association Executive Board charged the Commission on Practice to form a Task Force to 1.) review the existing occupational therapy terminology and relative value reporting systems, and 2.) develop a proposal for a national occupational therapy product reporting system.

At the time Public Law 95-142 was passed, no national system for reporting productivity of hospital-based occupational therapy services existed. The American Occupational Therapy Association Commission on Practice OT Uniform Reporting System Task Force was created in August 1978 to develop a proposal for a national system. Sylvia Harlock, OTR (Washington), member of the AOTA Commission on Practice, was appointed by the Commission Chair John Farace, OTR, to chair the Task Force.

Members selected to serve on the Task Force were:

Mary Lou Hymen, OTR	California
Kathy McFarland, OTR	Washington
Kathy Saunders, OTR	Wisconsin
Louise Thibodaux, OTR	Alabama
Carole Hays, OTR	Division on Practice, AOTA National Office

DESCRIPTION OF OCCUPATIONAL THERAPY SERVICE

Given the diversity of services provided by occupational therapy, the multiplicity of evaluation and treatment procedures which may often be used to achieve the same treatment outcomes, and the lack of a uniformly used description of occupational therapy service delivery, including definitions of terminology, the Task Force first developed the Description of Occupational Therapy Services. In selecting items and defining terms, the following criteria were taken into consideration:

1. Emphasis on description of treatment outcomes rather than treatment procedures.

2. Reflection of Medicare and Medicaid guidelines in terminology and category selection and definition.

3. Comprehensive description of occupational therapy services/product.

4. Reflection of the uniqueness of occupational therapy services/product in comparison with the services of other professions.

5. Coverage of recognized occupational therapy role in medical practice rather than all possible occupational therapy roles.

OCCUPATIONAL THERAPY FUNCTION

Occupational therapy is the application of purposeful, goal-oriented activity in the evaluation, problem identification, and/or treatment of persons whose function is impaired by physical illness or injury, emotional disorder, congenital or developmental disability, or the aging process, in order to achieve optimum functioning, to prevent disability, and to maintain health. Specific occupational therapy services include, but are not limited to, the following:

Education and training and evaluation of performance capacity in activities of daily living (ADL); the design, fabrication, and application of orthoses (splints); sensorimotor activities; guidance in selection and use of adaptive equipment; therapeutic use of activities and the activity process to develop/restore function performance; prevocational evaluation and training; consultation concerning the adaptation of physical environments for the handicapped; involvement in discharge planning and community re-entry; time/space/role management; and opportunity for self-expression and communication. These services are provided to individuals, groups, and to the community.

OCCUPATIONAL THERAPY SERVICES OUTLINE

I. Occupational Therapy Assessment
   A. Screening
   B. Patient-Related Consultation
   C. Evaluation
      1. Independent Living/Daily Living Skills and Performance
      2. Sensorimotor Skill and Performance Components
      3. Cognitive Skill and Performance Components

4. Psychosocial Skill and Performance Components

5. Therapeutic Adaptations

6. Specialized Evaluation

D. Reassessment

II. Occupational Therapy Treatment

  A. Independent Living/Daily Living Skills

    1. Physical Daily Living Skills

      a. Grooming and Hygiene

      b. Feeding/Eating

      c. Dressing

      d. Functional Mobility

      e. Functional Communication

      f. Object Manipulation

    2. Psychological/Emotional Daily Living Skills

      a. Self-Concept/Self-Identity

      b. Situational Coping

      c. Community Involvement

    3. Work

      a. Homemaking

      b. Child Care/Parenting

      c. Employment Preparation

    4. Play/Leisure

  B. Sensorimotor Components

    1. Neuromuscular

      a. Reflex Integration

      b. Range of Motion

      c. Gross and Fine Coordination

      d. Strength and Endurance

    2. Sensory Integration

      a. Sensory Awareness

      b. Visual-Spatial Awareness

      c. Body Integration

  C. Cognitive Components

    1. Orientation

    2. Conceptualization/Comprehension

      a. Concentration

      b. Attention Span

      c. Memory

    3. Cognitive Integration

      a. Generalization

      b. Problem Solving

  D. Psychosocial Components

    1. Self-Management

      a. Self-Expression

      b. Self-Control

    2. Dyadic Interaction

    3. Group Interaction

  E. Therapeutic Adaptation

    1. Orthotics

    2. Prosthetics

    3. Assistive/Adaptive Equipment

  F. Prevention

    1. Energy Conservation

    2. Joint Protection/Body Mechanics

3. Positioning

4. Coordination of Daily Living Activities

III. Patient/Client-Related Conferences

  A. Professional Conferences

  B. Agency Conferences

  C. Patient/Client-Advocate Conferences

IV. Travel: Patient-Treatment Related

The following items do not involve direct patient care.

V. Service Management

  A. Quality Review/Maintenance of Quality

    1. Development of Standards of Quality Treatment/Services

    2. Chart Audit

    3. Accrediting Reviews

    4. Occupational Therapy Care Review

    5. Inservice Education

  B. Departmental Maintenance

  C. Employee Meetings

  D. Program-Related Conferences

  E. Supervision

VI. Education

  A. Occupational Therapy Clinical Education: Occupational Therapy Students

  B. Occupational Therapy Clinical Education: Others

  C. Continuing Education

VII. Research

Occupational Therapy Services Description

I. Occupational Therapy Assessment

Occupational therapy assessment refers to the process of determining the need for, nature of, and estimated time of treatment, determining the needed coordination with other persons involved, and documenting these activities.

  A. Screening

Screening refers to the review of potential patient's/client's case to determine the need for evaluation and treatment. It includes discussion with other professionals and/or patient advocate, and patient/client interview or administration of screening tool.

  B. Patient-Related Consultation

Patient-related consultation refers to the sharing of relevant information with other professionals of patients/clients who are not currently referred to occupational therapy. This may include but is not limited to discussion, chart review, treatment recommendation, and documentation.

  C. Evaluation

Evaluation refers to the process of obtaining and interpreting data necessary for treatment. This includes planning for and documenting the evaluation process and results. This data may be gathered through record review, specific observation, interview, and the administration of data collection procedures. Such procedures include but are not limited to the use of standardized tests, performance checklists, and activities and tasks designed to evaluate specific performance abilities. Categories of occupational therapy evaluation include the independent living/daily living skills and performance and their components.

1. Independent Living/Daily Living Skills and Performance (see IIA).
2. Sensorimotor Skill and Performance Components (see IIB).
3. Cognitive Skill and Performance Components (see IIC).
4. Psychosocial Skill and Performance Components (see IID).
5. Therapeutic Adaptations (see IIE).
6. Specialized Evaluations

   Specialized evaluations refer to evaluations or tests requiring specialized training and/or advanced education to administer and interpret. Examples of specialized evaluations are employment preparation, evaluation (prevocational testing), sensory integration evaluation, prosthetic evaluation, driver's training evaluation.

D. Reassessment

Reassessment refers to the process of obtaining and interpreting data necessary for updating treatment plans and goals. This frequently involves administering only portions of the initial evaluation, documenting results, and/or revising treatment.

II. Occupational Therapy Treatment

Occupational therapy treatment refers to the use of specific activities or methods to develop, improve, and/or restore the performance of necessary functions; compensate for dysfunction and/or minimize debilitation; and the planning for and documenting of treatment performance. The necessary functions treated in occupational therapy are the following:

A. Independent Living/Daily Living Skills
1. Physical Daily Living Skills

   Physical daily living skills refer to the skill and performance of daily personal care, with or without adaptive equipment. It includes but is not limited to:

   a. Grooming and Hygiene

      Grooming and hygiene refer to the skill and performance of personal health needs, such as bathing, toileting, hair care, shaving, applying make-up.

   b. Feeding/Eating

      Feeding/eating refers to the skill and performance of sequentially feeding oneself, including sucking, chewing, swallowing, and using appropriate utensils.

   c. Dressing

      Dressing refers to the skill and performance of choosing appropriate clothing, dressing oneself in a sequential fashion, including fastening and adjusting clothing.

   d. Functional Mobility

      Functional mobility refers to the skill and performance in moving oneself from one position or place to another. It includes skills necessary for activities such as bed mobility, wheelchair mobility, transfers (bed, car, tub, toilet, chair), and functional ambulation, with or without adaptive aids. It also includes use of public and private travel systems, such as driving own automobile and using public transportation.

   e. Functional Communication

      Functional communication refers to the skill and performance in using equipment or systems to enhance or provide communication, such as writing equipment, typewriters, letterboards, telephone, Braille writers, artificial vocalization systems, and computers.

   f. Object Manipulation

      Object manipulation refers to the skill and performance in handling large and small common objects, such as calculators, keys, money, light switches, doorknobs, and packages.

2. Psychological/Emotional Daily Living Skills

   Psychological/emotional daily living skills refers to the skill and performance in developing one's self-concept/self-identity, coping with life situations, and participating in one's organizational and community environment. It includes but is not limited to:

   a. Self-Concept/Self-Identity

      Self-concept/self-identity refers to the cognitive image of one's functional self. This includes but is not limited to:

      (1) Clearly perceiving one's needs, feelings, conflicts, values, beliefs, expectations, sexuality, and power.

      (2) Realistically perceiving one's needs, feelings, conflicts, values, beliefs, expectations, sexuality, and power.

      (3) Knowing one's performance strengths and limitations.

      (4) Sensing one's competence, achievement, self-esteem, and self-respect.

      (5) Integrating new experiences with established self-concept/self-identity.

      (6) Having a sense of psychological safety and security.

      (7) Perceiving one's goals and directions.

   b. Situational Coping

      Situational coping refers to skill and performance in handling stress and dealing with problems and changes in a manner that is functional for self and others. This includes but is not limited to:

      (1) Setting goals, selecting, harmonizing, and managing activities of daily living to promote optimal performance.

      (2) Testing goals and perceptions against reality.

      (3) Perceiving changes and need for changes in self and environment.

      (4) Directing and redirecting energy to overcome problems.

      (5) Initiating, implementing, and following through on decisions.

      (6) Assuming responsibility for self and consequences of actions.

      (7) Interacting with others, dyadic and group.

   c. Community Involvement

      Community involvement refers to skill and performance in interacting within one's social system. This includes but is not limited to:

      (1) Understanding social norms and their impact on society.

      (2) Planning, organizing, and executing daily life activities in relationship to society, including such activities as budgeting, time management, social role management, arranging for housing, nutritional planning, assessing and using community resources.

      (3) Recognizing and responding to needs to families, groups, and complex social units.

      (4) Understanding and responding to organizational/

community role expectations as both recipient and contributor.

3. Work

Work refers to skill and performance in participating in socially purposeful and productive activities. These activities may take place in the home, employment setting, school, or community. They include but are not limited to:

a. Homemaking

Homemaking refers to skill and performance in homemaking and home management tasks, such as meal planning, meal preparation and clean-up, laundry, cleaning, minor household repairs, shopping, and use of household safety principles.

b. Child Care/Parenting

Child care/parenting refers to skill and performance in child care activities and management. This includes but is not limited to physical care of children, and use of age-appropriate activities, communication, and behavior to facilitate child development.

c. Employment Preparation

Employment preparation refers to skill and performance in precursory job activities (including prevocational activities). This includes but is not limited to:

(1) Job acquisition skills and performance.

(2) Organizational and team participatory skills and performance.

(3) Work process skills and performance.

(4) Work product quality.

4. Play/Leisure

Play/leisure refers to skill and performance in choosing, performing, and engaging in activities for amusement, relaxation, spontaneous enjoyment, and/or self-expression. This includes but is not limited to:

a. Recognizing one's specific needs, interests, and adaptations necessary for performance.

b. Identifying characteristics of activities and social situations that make them play for the individual.

c. Identifying activities that contain those characteristics.

d. Choosing play activities for participation, such as sports, games, hobbies, music, drama, and other activities.

e. Testing out and adapting activities to enable participation.

f. Identifying and using community resources.

B. Sensorimotor Components

Sensorimotor components refer to the skill and performance of patterns of sensory and motor behavior that are prerequisites to self-care, work, and play/leisure performance. The components in this section include neuromuscular and sensory integrative skills, including perceptual motor skills.

1. Neuromuscular

Neuromuscular refers to the skill and performance of motor aspects of behavior. This includes but is not limited to:

a. Reflex Integration

Reflex integration refers to skill and performance in enhancing and supporting functional neuromuscular development through eliciting and/or inhibiting stereotyped, patterned, and/or involuntary responses coordinated at subcortical and cortical levels.

b. Range of Motion

Range of motion refers to skill and performance in using maximum span of joint movement in activities with and without assistance to enhance functional performance. The standard levels of performance include:

(1) Active range of motion: movement by patient, unassisted through a complete range of motion.

(2) Passive range of motion: movement performed by someone other than patient or by a mechanical device, requiring no muscle contraction on the part of the patient.

(3) Active-assistive range of motion: movement performed by the patient to the limit of his/her ability, and then completed with assistance.

c. Gross and Fine Coordination

Gross and fine coordination refers to skill and performance in muscle control, coordination, and dexterity while participating in activities.

(1) Muscle control: refers to skill and performance in directing muscle movement.

(2) Coordination: refers to skill and performance in gross motor activities using several muscle groups.

(3) Dexterity: refers to skill and performance in tasks using small muscle groups.

d. Strength and Endurance

Strength and endurance refers to skill and performance in using muscular force within time periods necessary for purposeful task performance. This involves but is not limited to progressively building strength and cardia and pulmonary reserve, increasing the length of work periods, and decreasing fatigue and strain.

2. Sensory Integration

Sensory integration refers to skill and performance in development and coordination of sensory input, motor output, and sensory feedback. This includes but is not limited to:

a. Sensory Awareness

Sensory awareness refers to skill and performance in perceiving and differentiating external and internal stimuli, such as:

(1) Tactile awareness: the perception and interpretation of stimuli through skin contact.

(2) Stereognosis: the identification of forms and nature of objects through the sense of touch.

(3) Kinesthesia: the conscious perception of muscular motion, weight, and position.

(4) Proprioceptive awareness: the identification of the positions of body parts in space.

(5) Ocular control: the localization and visual tracking of stimuli.

(6) Vestibular awareness: the detention of motion and gravitational pull as related to one's performance in functional activities, ambulation, and balance.

(7) Auditory awareness: the differentiation and identification of sounds.

(8) Gustatory awareness: the differentiation and identification of tastes.

(9) Olfactory awareness: the differentiation and identification of smells.

b. Visual-Spatial Awareness

Visual-spatial awareness refers to skill and performance in perceiving distances between and relationships among objects, including self. This includes but is not limited to:

(1) Figure-ground: recognition of forms and objects when presented in a configuration with competing stimuli.

(2) Form constancy: recognition of forms and objects as the same when presented in different contexts.

(3) Position in space: knowledge of one's position in space relative to other objects.

  c. Body Integration

Body integration refers to skill and performance in perceiving and regulating the position of various muscles and body parts in relationship to each other during static and movement states. This includes but is not limited to:

(1) Body schema: refers to the perception of one's physical self through proprioceptive and interoceptive sensations.

(2) Postural balance: refers to skill and performance in developing and maintaining body posture while sitting, standing, or engaging in activity.

(3) Bilateral motor coordination: refers to skill and performance in purpose.

(4) Right-left discrimination: refers to skill and performance in differentiating right from left and vice versa.

(5) Visual-motor integration: refers to skill and performance in combining visual input with purposeful voluntary movement of the hand and other body parts involved in an activity. Visual-motor integration includes eye-hand coordination.

(6) Crossing the midline: refers to skill and performance in crossing the vertical midline of the body.

(7) Praxis: refers to skill and performance of purposeful movement that involves motor planning.

C. Cognitive Components

Cognitive components refer to skill and performance of the mental processes necessary to know or apprehend by understanding. This includes but is not limited to:

1. Orientation

Orientation refers to skill and performance in comprehending, defining, and adjusting oneself in an environment with regard to time, place, and person.

2. Conceptualization/Comprehension

Conceptualization/comprehension refers to skill and performance in conceiving and understanding concepts or tasks such as color identification, word recognition, sign concepts, sequencing, matching, association, classification, and abstracting. This includes but is not limited to:

  a. Concentration

Concentration refers to skill and performance in focusing on a designated task or concept.

  b. Attention Span

Attention span refers to skill and performance in focusing on a task or concept for a particular length of time.

  c. Memory

Memory refers to skill and performance in retaining and recalling tasks or concepts from the past.

3. Cognitive Integration

Cognitive integration refers to skill and performance in applying diverse knowledge to environmental situations. This involves but is not limited to:

  a. Generalization

Generalization refers to skill and performance in applying specific concepts to a variety of related situations.

  b. Problem Solving

Problem solving refers to skill and performance in identifying and organizing solutions to difficulties. It includes but is not limited to:

(1) Defining or evaluating the problem.

(2) Organizing a plan.

(3) Making decisions/judgments.

(4) Implementing plan, including following through in logical sequence.

(5) Evaluating decision/judgment and plan.

D. Psychosocial Components

Psychosocial components refer to skill and performance in self-management, dyadic and group interaction.

1. Self-Management

Self-management refers to skill and performance in expressing and controlling oneself in functional and creative activities.

  a. Self-Expression

Self-expression refers to skill and performance in perceiving one's feelings and interpreting and using a variety of communication signs and symbols. This includes but is not limited to:

(1) Experiencing and recognizing a range of emotions.

(2) Having an adequate vocabulary.

(3) Having writing and speaking skills.

(4) Interpreting and using correctly an adequate range of nonverbal signs and symbols.

  b. Self-Control

Self-control refers to skill and performance in modulating and modifying present behaviors, and in initiating new behaviors in accordance with situational demands. It includes but is not limited to:

(1) Observing own and other's behavior.

(2) Conceptualizing problems in terms of needed behavioral changes or action.

(3) Imitating new behaviors.

(4) Directing and redirecting energies into stress-reducing activities and behaviors.

2. Dyadic Interaction

Dyadic interaction refers to skill and performance in relating to another person. This includes but is not limited to:

  a. Understanding social/cultural norms of communication and interaction in various activity and social situations.

  b. Setting limits on self and others.

  c. Compromising and negotiating.

  d. Handling competition, frustration, anxiety, success, and failure.

  e. Cooperating and competing with others.

  f. Responsibly relying on self and others.

3. Group Interaction

Group interaction refers to skill and performance in relating to groups of three to six persons, or larger. This includes but is not limited to:

a. Knowing and performing a variety of task and social/emotional role behaviors.

b. Understanding common stages of group process.

c. Participating in a group in a manner that is mutually beneficial to self and others.

E. Therapeutic Adaptation

Therapeutic adaptations refer to the design and/or restructuring of the physical environment to assist self-care, work, and play/leisure performance. This includes selecting, obtaining, fitting and fabricating equipment, and instructing the client, family and/or staff in proper use and care of equipment. It also includes minor repair and modification for correct fit, position, or use. Categories of therapeutic adaptations consist of:

1. Orthotics

Orthotics refer to the provision of dynamic and static splints, braces, and slings for the purpose of relieving pain, maintaining joint alignment, protecting joint integrity, improving function, and/or decreasing deformity.

2. Prosthetics

Prosthetics refer to the training in use of artificial substitutes of missing body parts, which augment performance of function.

3. Assistive/Adaptive Equipment

Assistive/adaptive equipment refers to the provision of special devices that assist in performance and/or structural or positional changes such as the installation of ramps, bars, changes in furniture heights, adjustments of traffic patterns, and modifications of wheelchairs.

F. Prevention

Prevention refers to skill and performance in minimizing debilitation. It may include programs for persons where predisposition to disability exists, as well as for those who have already incurred a disability. This includes but is not limited to:

1. Energy Conservation

Energy conservation refers to skill and performance in applying energy-saving procedures, activity restriction, work simplification, time management, and/or organization of the environment to minimize energy output.

2. Joint Protection/Body Mechanics

Joint protection/body mechanics refers to skill and performance in applying principles or procedures to minimize stress on joints. Procedures may include the use of proper body mechanics, avoidance of static or deforming postures, and/or avoidance of excessive weight-bearing.

3. Positioning

Positioning refers to skill and performance in the placement of a body part in alignment to promote optimal functioning.

4. Coordination of Daily Living Activities

Coordination of daily living activities refers to skill and performance in selecting and coordinating activities of self-care, work, play/leisure, and rest to promote optimal performance of daily life tasks.

III. Patient/Client-Related Conferences

Patient/client-related conferences include participating in meetings to discuss and identify needs, treatment program, and future plans of referred client and documenting such participation. Patient/client may or may not be present. Categories of conferences include:

A. Professional Conferences

Professional conferences refer to participating in meetings with a group or individual professionals to discuss patient's/client's status, and to advise/consult regarding treatment needs. Synonymous terms for professional conferences include initial conference, interim review, discharge planning, case conference, and others.

B. Agency Conferences

Agency conferences refer to participating in meetings with vocational, social, religious, recreational health, educational, and other community representatives to assess, implement, or coordinate the use of services.

C. Patient/Client-Advocate Conferences

Patient/client-advocate conferences refer to participating in meetings with client advocate (e.g., family, guardian, or others responsible for patient/client) to assess patient's/client's situation, set goals, plan treatment and/or discharge; and/or to instruct client advocate to support or carry out treatment program.

IV. Travel: Patient-Treatment Related

Travel: patient-treatment related refers to travel by therapists, with or without patient; that is, related to direct patient treatment.

Commission on Practice, the American Occupational Therapy Association, Inc.

Adopted March 1979 by the Representative Assembly, AOTA.

Appendix C

Blank Student Worksheets

FORM 1
ACTIVITY AWARENESS FORM

Student: _____ Date: _____
Activity: _____
Course: _____

Directions: Reflecting on the activity just performed, complete the following sentences with the first words that come to mind.

1. During this activity I was thinking about…

2. While doing this activity I felt…

3. In doing this activity, the parts of my body I remember using were…

4. To do this activity I need to (mentally, emotionally, physically)…

5. When I do this activity again I will…

6. From doing this activity I became aware of…

FORM 2
ACTION IDENTIFICATION FORM

Student: _____   Date: _____
Activity: _____
Course: _____

Directions: Select an activity, and using the Do-What-How style, list the major actions (in sequence in 10 steps or less) required for you to perform this activity. Repeat the exercise after observing someone else perform the same activity.

Observation of Self

Observation of Another

FORM 3
ACTIVITY ANALYSIS FOR EXPECTED PERFORMANCE

Student: _____   Date: _____

Activity: _____

Course: _____

Section 1: Activity Summary

Directions: Respond to the following in list format.

A. Name and Brief Description of Activity

B. Sequence of Major Steps (in 10 steps or less; specify time required to complete each step)

C. Precautions (review "Sequence of Major Steps")

D. Special Considerations (age appropriateness, educational requirements, cultural relevance, gender identification, other)

E. Acceptable Criteria for Completed Activity

F. Activity Demands
   1. Objects and Their Properties (tools, materials, equipment, inherent properties)

   2. Space Demands (size, arrangement, surface, lighting, temperature, noise, humidity, ventilation)

   3. Social Demands

Section 2: Analyzing Performance Areas of Occupation

A. Activities of Daily Living (ADL)
   1. Bathing, Showering

   2. Bowel and Bladder Management

   3. Dressing

   4. Eating

   5. Feeding

   6. Functional Mobility

   7. Personal Device Care

FORM 3
ACTIVITY ANALYSIS FOR EXPECTED PERFORMANCE (CONTINUED)

8. Personal Hygiene and Grooming

9. Sexual Activity

10. Sleep/Rest

11. Toilet Hygiene

B. Instrumental Activities of Daily Living (IADL)
   1. Care of Others

   2. Care of Pets

   3. Child Rearing

   4. Communication Device Use

   5. Community Mobility

   6. Financial Management

   7. Health Management and Maintenance

   8. Home Establishment and Management

   9. Meal Preparation and Cleanup

   10. Safety Procedures and Emergency Response

   11. Shopping

C. Education
   1. Formal Educational Participation

   2. Exploration of Informal Personal Educational Needs or Interests

   3. Informal Personal Education Preparation

D. Work
   1. Employment Interest and Pursuits

   2. Employment Seeking and Acquisition

FORM 3
ACTIVITY ANALYSIS FOR EXPECTED PERFORMANCE (CONTINUED)

    3. Job Performance

    4. Retirement Preparation and Adjustment

    5. Volunteer Exploration

    6. Volunteer Participation

E. Play
    1. Play Exploration

    2. Play Participation

F. Leisure
    1. Leisure Exploration

    2. Leisure Participation

G. Social Participation
    1. Community

    2. Family

    3. Peer, Friend

Section 3: Analyzing Performance Skills and Client Factors

Part I. Performance Skills
A. Motor Skills
    1. Posture (stabilizes, aligns, positions)

    2. Mobility (walks, reaches, bends)

    3. Coordination (coordinates, manipulates, flows)

    4. Strength and Effort (moves, transports, lifts, calibrates, grips)

    5. Energy (endures, paces)

FORM 3
ACTIVITY ANALYSIS FOR EXPECTED PERFORMANCE (CONTINUED)

B. Process skills

   1. Energy (paces, attends)

   2. Knowledge (chooses, uses, handles, heeds, inquires)

   3. Temporal Organization (initiates, continues, sequences, terminates)

   4. Organizing Space and Objects (searches/locates, gathers, organizes, restores, navigates)

   5. Adaptation (notices/responds, accommodates, adjusts, benefits)

C. Communication/Interaction Skills

   1. Physicality (contacts, gazes, gestures, maneuvers, orients, postures)

   2. Information Exchange (articulates, asserts, asks, engages, expresses, modulates, shares, speaks, sustains)

   3. Relations (collaborates, conforms, focuses, relates, respects)

Part II. Client Factors

A. Body Function Categories

   1. Mental Functions (affective, cognitive, perceptual)

     a. Global (consciousness, orientation, sleep, temperament and personality, energy and drive)

     b. Specific (attention, memory, perceptual, thought, higher-level cognition, language, calculation, motor planning, psychomotor, emotional, experience of self and time)

   2. Sensory Functions and Pain

     a. Seeing

     b. Hearing/Vestibular

     c. Other (taste, smell, proprioception, touch, discrimination)

     d. Pain

   3. Neuromusculoskeletal and Movement-Related Functions

     a. Joints and Bones (mobility, stability)

     b. Muscle (power, tone, endurance)

     c. Movement (motor reflex, reactions, voluntary, involuntary, gait)

FORM 3
ACTIVITY ANALYSIS FOR EXPECTED PERFORMANCE (CONTINUED)

    d. Cardiovascular, Hematological, Immunological, and Respiratory

    e. Voice and Speech

    f. Digestive, Metabolic, and Endocrine

    g. Genitourinary and Reproductive

    h. Skin, Hair, and Nails

B. Body Structure Categories
1. Nervous System

2. Eye, Ear, and Related Structures

3. Voice and Speech

4. Cardiovascular, Immunological, and Respiratory

5. Digestive

6. Genitourinary and Reproductive

7. Movement

8. Skin and Related Structures

Section 4: Analyzing Performance Patterns and Contexts

Part I. Performance Patterns
A. Habits
1. Useful

2. Impoverished

3. Dominating

B. Routines

C. Roles

FORM 3
ACTIVITY ANALYSIS FOR EXPECTED PERFORMANCE (CONTINUED)

Part II. Performance Contexts

A. Cultural

B. Physical

C. Social

D. Personal

E. Spiritual

F. Temporal

G. Virtual

FORM 4
ACTIVITY ANALYSIS FOR THERAPEUTIC INTERVENTION

Student: _____ Date: _____

Activity: _____

Course: _____

Section 1: Activity Description

A. Provide a Brief Description of Activity

B. Identify Major Steps

Section 2: Therapeutic Qualities

A. Energy Patterns—Describe the required energy level in terms of light, moderate, or heavy work patterns and provide an explanation for the level specified (refer to description of MET levels in Unit 6). Consider the client factors of the cardiovascular and respiratory systems as well as muscle endurance.

B. Activity Patterns—Indicate the patterns of the activity expected for successful completion of the activity.
   1. Structural/Methodical/Orderly

   2. Repetitive

   3. Expressive/Creative/Projective

   4. Tactile
      a. Contact With Others (e.g., hands-on, stand by assist)

      b. Materials (pliable, sensual)

      c. Equipment (e.g., size, manageability, shape)

C. Performance Patterns
   1. Habits (useful, impoverished, dominating)

   2. Routines

   3. Roles

FORM 4
ACTIVITY ANALYSIS FOR THERAPEUTIC INTERVENTION (CONTINUED)

Section 3: Therapeutic Application

A. Population—Discuss for whom and in what way increased occupational performance can be derived from the use of this activity. Consider performance skills for motor, process, and communication/interaction. Identify any contraindications.

B. Gradation—Describe ways to grade this activity in terms of:
1. Activity Sequence, Duration, and/or the Activity Procedures

2. Working Position of the Individual

3. Tools
   a. Position

   b. Size

   c. Shape

   d. Weight

   e. Texture

4. Materials
   a. Position

   b. Size

   c. Shape

   d. Weight

   e. Texture

5. Nature/Degree of Interpersonal Contact

6. Extent of Tactile, Verbal, or Visual Cues Used by Practitioner During Activity

7. The Teaching-Learning Environment

FORM 4
ACTIVITY ANALYSIS FOR THERAPEUTIC INTERVENTION (CONTINUED)

C. Therapeutic Modifications—Indicate ways in which this activity may be changed to increase occupational performance. State your reasoning. Write n/a if not applicable. Definitions for the following terms can be found in Appendix B, *Uniform Terminology for Reporting Occupational Therapy Service, First Edition*, "Therapeutic Adaptations" and *The Guide to Occupational Therapy Practice* (AOTA, 1999).

1. Therapeutic Adaptations
   a. Orthotic Devices

   b. Prosthetic Devices

   c. Assistive Technology and Adaptive Devices
      (1) Architectural Modification

      (2) Environmental Modification

      (3) Tool and Equipment Modification (low-tech [e.g., reacher] or hi-tech [e.g., computer control devices])

      (4) Wheelchair Modification

2. Prevention
   a. Energy Conservation
      (1) Energy-Saving Procedures

      (2) Activity Restriction

      (3) Work Simplification

      (4) Time Management

      (5) Environmental Organization

   b. Joint Protection/Body Mechanics
      (1) Using Proper Body Mechanics

      (2) Avoiding Static/Deforming Postures

      (3) Avoiding Excessive Weight-Bearing

   c. Positioning

FORM 4

ACTIVITY ANALYSIS FOR THERAPEUTIC INTERVENTION (CONTINUED)

d. Balance of Performance Areas to Facilitate Health and Well-Being

    (1) Enhancement of Occupational Performance Areas

    (2) Satisfaction of Client and/or Caregiver

    (3) Quality of Life

FORM 5
CLIENT-ACTIVITY INTERVENTION PLAN

Student: _____ Date: _____

Activity: _____

Course: _____

1. Client Occupational Profile and Referral
    A. Client Occupational Profile

    B. Referral

2. Intervention Goals
    A. Long-Term Goal (First Priority)

    B. Short-Term Goal (Support)

3. Intervention Activity Description

4. Intervention Activity Preparation
    A. Review Goals and Describe Practitioner's Role

    B. Personnel Required to Complete the Preparation

    C. Required Preparation Time

    D. Required Place and Space

    E. Materials

FORM 5
CLIENT-ACTIVITY INTERVENTION PLAN (CONTINUED)

F. Equipment

G. Safety Precautions for Personnel

5. Intervention Activity Implementation
   A. Personnel

   B. Setting and Location

   C. Space Required

   D. Environment

   E. Materials

   F. Equipment: Assistive Devices and Adaptations Included

   G. Required Intervention Time

   H. Safety Precautions for Client

6. Intervention Activity Sequence (10 action steps or less)

7. Documentation:
   A. Domain

   B. Process

Index

accountability, 88
action, 37
action identification, 25, 35–37
Action Identification Form, 39, 101
    blank worksheet, 159
    directions for, 37
    objectives of, 37
activities of daily living (ADL), 7, 18, 20, 21
    in activity analysis, 46
    analysis of, 103–104
    coordination of, 154
activity
    adaptation of, 65–66
    assumptions about, 35–36
    breaking into small units, 64
    definition of, 16, 35
    description of, 73, 75, 116
        in Activity Analysis for Therapeutic Intervention, 110
        in Client-Activity Intervention Plan, 87
    dynamic quality of, 35
    focus on, 17
    gradation of, 63–65, 66, 144
    heritage of, 15–16
    identifying components of, 37
    implementation of, 117–118
        in Client-Activity Intervention Plan, 88
    performance of, 97
    preparation of, 116–117
        in Client-Activity Intervention Plan, 87–88
    purposeful, 16, 24, 125–126, 142, 144
    sequence of, 118
        in Client-Activity Intervention Plan, 88
    summary of, in Activity Analysis for Expected Performance, 102–103
    versatility of, 97
activity analysis, 8, 15–25, 125
    application of, 125–126
    core of, 23
    for expected performance, 45–55
    learning approach for, 23–24
    multilevel approach to, 24–25
    process of, 88
        rationale for, 18–23
    for therapeutic intervention, 73–74

Activity Analysis for Expected Performance Form, 102–109
    activity summary section of, 45, 48–49
    analyzing performance areas of occupation section of, 45, 49–51
    analyzing performance patterns and contexts in, 46, 54–55
    analyzing performance skills and client factors section in, 46, 51–54
    blank worksheet, 160–165
Activity Analysis for Therapeutic Intervention Form, 110–115
    activity description section of, 73, 75
    blank worksheet, 166–169
    therapeutic application section of, 74, 76–79
    therapeutic qualities section of, 73, 75–76
activity awareness, 24, 35–37
Activity Awareness Form, 38, 100
    blank worksheet, 158
    directions for, 36
    objective of, 36
adaptation, 65–66, 144, 154
    definition of, 65
    examples of, 65
    therapeutic, 113–115
adaptive devices, 113–114
adaptive equipment, 154
adaptive occupation, 6
ADL. See activities of daily living (ADL)
adverb, descriptive qualities of, 37
agency conferences, 154
American Occupational Therapy Association (AOTA)
    Commission on Practice OT Uniform Reporting System Task Force of, 149
    on occupation, 6
    position papers of, 141–147
AOTA (American Occupational Therapy Association). See American Occupational Therapy Association (AOTA)
assistive equipment, 154
assistive technology, 66, 113–114
    utilizing, 123
attention span, 153
auditory awareness, 152

body function, 20
    analyzing, 107–108
    categories of, 22

body integration, 153
body mechanics, 114, 154
body schema, 153
body structures, 20
    categories of, 22
        analysis of, 108–109

cardiac rehabilitation, graded exercise in, 64
caregiver satisfaction, 115
case study, 88
child care skills, 152
children with physical disabilities, planning for, 147
client-activity intervention plan, 8, 25, 85
    activity description in, 87
    activity implementation in, 88
    activity preparation in, 87–88
    activity sequence in, 88
    case study of, 86–87
    documentation of, 88–89
    goals of, 85–86, 87
    occupational profile in, 87
Client-Activity Intervention Plan Form, 87, 90–92, 116–118
    blank worksheet, 170–171
client-advocate conferences, 154
client factors, 19–20
    analysis of, 46, 52–54
        in Activity Analysis for Expected Performance, 107–109
    description of, 22
client satisfaction, 115
clinical reasoning process, 23, 87, 125
cognitive integration, 153
cognitive skills, 153
communication/interaction skills, 20, 21
    analysis of, 107
community
    health of, 126
    involvement in, 151–152
compensatory occupation, 6
comprehension, 153
compromise, 153
concentration, 153
conceptualization/comprehension skills, 153
conditional reasoning, 23
contrived occupation, 6
coordination, 152
cost containment, 88
cultural context, 20, 22

daily living activities. *See* activities of daily living (ADL)
deficits, impact of, 25
Dewey, John, 141
dexterity, 152
disability
    dimensions of, 17
    life roles before, 8
    state of inactivity and, 36
Do-What-How style, 37
documentation
    domain, 88, 118
    process, 88–89, 118

doing, 37, 146
    process of, 35
domain, documentation of, 88, 118
dressing
    in ADL performance, 18
    skills in, 151
dyadic interaction, 153

education, 20, 21
educational programs, 23–24
Eleanor Clarke Slagle Lectureship recipients, writings of, 126
employment preparation, 152
endurance data, 73
endurance skills, 152
energy conservation, 154
    modifications for, 114
energy needs, for activities, 64
environmental organization, 114
ergonomics, development of, 66
evaluation, 150–151
evaluation tools, 8
exercise, 6
expected performance, activity analysis of, 25, 45–55, 102–109

feeding/eating skills, 151
fine motor coordination, 152
forms
    blank, 158–171
    Web site for, 123
function, 142
    definition of, 146
functional assessment, 8
functional communication, 151
functional mobility, 151
functional outcomes, 7

generalization, 153
gradation, 112–113
    of activities, 63–65, 66, 144
    realistic, 66
grading. *See* gradation
grooming, 151
gross coordination, 152
group interaction, 153–154

habits, 20, 22
health
    activity and, 36
    continuum of, 36
    promotion of, 16–17
Henry Phipps Clinic, 6
homemaking, 152
hygiene, 151

IADL. *See* instrumental activities of daily living (IADL)
in-home kitchen experience, 6
inactivity, disability and, 36
Independent Daily Living Skills, 151–152
instrumental activities of daily living (IADL), 20, 21
    analysis of, 104–105

interactive reasoning, 23
International Classification of Functioning, Disability, and Health (WHO), 17
intervention
 methods of, 6
 true-life experiences as strategies of, 6
intervention goals
 in Client-Activity Intervention Plan, 87
 long-term, 88, 116
 short-term, 88, 116

James, William, 141
joint protection, 154
 modifications for, 114–115

kinesthesia, 152

learning approach, 23–24
learning process, activity analysis in, 15–25
leisure, 7, 20, 21, 152
life roles, 8
lifestyle, constructing, 35
limit setting, 153

memory, 153
metabolic equivalent units (METs), 73
Meyer, Adolph, 15, 35, 141
midline, crossing, 153
Model Definition of Occupational Therapy Practice for the AOTA Model Practice Act, revision of, 17–18
motion analysis, 23
motor coordination, bilateral, 153
motor skills, 20, 21
 analysis of, 106
muscle control, 152
mutual partnership, 8

negotiating, 153
nesting, 142
neuromuscular skills, 152
normal function, 16

object manipulation skills, 151
occupation
 applying to intervention programs, 16
 categories of, 142
 definition of, 6, 16, 141–142
 dimensions of, 142
 dynamic, multidimensional nature of, 141
 health-enhancing nature of, 45
 impact of on human experience, 5–8
 multidimensional meanings of, 15–16
 need for, 5, 16–17
 paradigm of, 7
 performance areas of, 19–20
 performance dimension of, 141
 position paper on, 141–142
 versus purposeful activity, 16
 reality of, 6

research on, 142
 study of, 142
 therapeutic benefits of, 142
occupational competence, progression toward, 7
occupational history, in activity grading, 65
occupational needs, 8
occupational performance, 88
 position paper on, 146–147
occupational performance areas
 major categories for, 20
occupational profile, 88, 116
 in Client-Activity Intervention Plan, 87
occupational science concepts, 7
occupational therapy
 activity analysis in, 125
 activity gradation in, 63–65
 adaptation in, 65–66
 definition of, 16
 goals of, 87–88
 heritage of, 15–16
 language of, 17–18, 19
 literature on, 6–7
 motion analysis in, 23
 versus physical therapy, 7
 position papers on, 16–17
 research on, 142
occupational therapy assessment, 149–150
 description of, 150–151
occupational therapy education, 144
occupational therapy function, 149
occupational therapy intervention, case study of, 88
Occupational Therapy Intervention Process Model, 8
Occupational Therapy Practice Framework, 125
 in activity analysis, 24
 adoption of, 7
 diagrammatic representation of, 18–22
 goals in, 88
 revised, 17
 second stage of, 87
Occupational Therapy Process, 87
occupational therapy scholars, 141
occupational therapy services
 description of, 149, 150–154
 outline of, 149–150
occupational therapy treatment, 150
 description of, 151–154
ocular control, 152
olfactory awareness, 152
on-the-job training, 6
orientation, 153
orthotic devices, 113, 154

parenting skills, 152
participation
 engagement to support, 19–20
 focus on, 17
patient/client-related conferences, 150, 154
patient-related consultation, 150
patient-treatment related travel, 154

Performance Area of Occupation, Activities of Daily Living, 18
performance areas, 21–22
    analysis of, 45, 49–51
        in Activity Analysis for Expected Performance, 103–105
performance contexts, 18, 19–20, 22
    in Activity Analysis for Expected Performance, 109
    analysis of, 46, 54–55
performance patterns, 19–20, 22
    analysis of, 46, 54–55, 109
performance skills, 19–20, 21
    analysis of, 46, 51–52, 106–107
Performances Areas, Uniform Terminology, 7
person-environment interactions model, 147
personal context, 20, 22
physical context, 20, 22
physical daily living skills, 151
physical disabilities, children with, 147
physical therapy, 7
play, 7, 20, 21, 152
position papers
    on occupation, 15–16
positioning, 154
positioning modifications, 115
postural balance, 153
Practice Act, 16–17
praxis, 153
prevention skills, 154
prioritizing, 64
problem solving, 153
procedural reasoning, 23
process
    documentation of, 88–89, 118
    review of, 100–118
process skills, 20, 21
    analysis of, 106–107
productive activities, 7
professional conferences, 154
professional performance, grading and adapting, 66
proprioceptive awareness, 152
prosthetic devices, 113, 154
psychological/emotional daily living skills, 151–152
psychosocial skills, 153–154
purposeful activity, 16, 126
    analysis of, 24
    definition of, 142
    position paper on, 144
    therapeutic use of, 125

quality of life, 115

range of motion, 152
real-life experiences, as intervention strategies, 6
reassessment, 151
reflex integration, 152
rehabilitation services, after world wars, 7
repetitions, for activity, 64
right-left discrimination, 153

roles, 20, 22
routines, 20, 22

screening, 150
self, observation of, 39, 101
self-actualization, 7
self-concept/self-identity, 151
self-control, 153
self-expression, 153
self-management, 153
sensorimotor skills, 152–153
sensory awareness, 152
sensory integration, 152–153
sickness, definition of, 36
situational coping, 151
Slagle, Eleanor Clarke, 141
    persona of, 6
social context, 20, 22
social/cultural norms, 153
social/emotional role behaviors, 154
social participation, 20, 21
specialized evaluation, 151
spiritual context, 20, 22
stereognosis, 152
strength skills, 152
student worksheets, blank, 158–171

tactile awareness, 152
Teaching Improvement Project System for Health Care Educators (TIPS), 37
telephoning skills, grading, 64
temporal context, 20, 22
therapeutic adaptation, 154
therapeutic application, 74, 76–79
    in Activity Analysis for Therapeutic Intervention, 111–115
therapeutic intervention, activity analysis for, 25, 73–74, 110–115
therapeutic modifications, 113–115
therapeutic occupation, 6
therapeutic purposes, 125
therapeutic qualities, 73, 75–76
    in Activity Analysis for Therapeutic Intervention, 110–111
therapeutic work, definition of, 15
therapist-imposed interventions, 6
thinking, modes of, 23
time management, 114
TIPS. *See Teaching Improvement Project System for Health Care Educators* (TIPS)
tool modification, 114
top-down approach, 8
travel skills, 154

Uniform Terminology, 125
    in activity analysis, 24
Uniform Terminology for Reporting Occupational Therapy Services
    First Edition, 149–154
    Third Edition, 7, 141–142
    revision of, 17

vestibular awareness, 152
virtual context, 20, 22
visual-motor integration, 153
visual-spatial awareness, 152–153

Web site, forms on, 123
well-being, activity and, 36
wheelchair modifications, 114

work, 7, 20, 21
work simplification, 114
work skills, 152

Yerxa, E., 5

WAIT

...There's More!

Please visit
www.slackbooks.com
to order any of these titles!
24 Hours a Day...7 Days a Week!

Attention Industry Partners!
Whether you are interested in buying multiple copies of a book, chapter reprints, or looking for something new and different — we are able to accommodate your needs.

Multiple Copies
At attractive discounts starting for purchases as low as 25 copies for a single title, SLACK Incorporated will be able to meet all your of your needs.

Chapter Reprints
SLACK Incorporated is able to offer the chapters you want in a format that will lead to success. Bound with an attractive cover, use the chapters that are a fit specifically for your company. Available for quantities of 100 or more.

Customize
SLACK Incorporated is able to create a specialized custom version of any of our products specifically for your company.

Please contact the Marketing Manager of the Professional Book Division for further details on multiple copy purchases, chapter reprints or custom printing at 1-800-257-8290 or 1-856-848-1000.

*Please note all conditions are subject to change.

CODE: 328

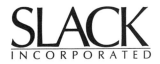

SLACK Incorporated • Professional Book Division
6900 Grove Road • Thorofare, NJ 08086
1-800-257-8290 or 1-856-848-1000
Fax: 1-856-853-5991 • E-mail: orders@slackinc.com • Visit: www.slackbooks.com